Soft Exercise

The Complete Book of Stretching

ARTHUR BALASKAS AND JOHN STIRK

Drawings by Candy Amsden

London
UNWIN PAPERBACKS
Boston   Sydney

First published in Great Britain by Unwin Paperbacks 1983
Reprinted 1983, 1984

UNWIN® PAPERBACKS
40 Museum Street, London WC1A 1LU, UK

Unwin Paperbacks,
Park Lane, Hemel Hempstead, Herts HP2 4TE, UK

George Allen & Unwin Australia Pty Ltd.,
8 Napier Street, North Sydney, NSW 2060, Australia

British Library Cataloguing in Publication Data

Balaskas, Arthur
   Soft exercise.
1. Exercise   2. Stretch (Physiology)
I. Title   II. Stirk, John
613.7'1   RA781
ISBN 0-04-513047-0

Set in 10 on 11pt Times by
Computape (Pickering) Ltd, North Yorkshire
and printed in Hong Kong by
Dah Hua Printing Press Co., Ltd.

A fit healthy body has strength and stamina, suppleness and stability. Hard exercise develops strength and stamina while soft exercise develops suppleness and stability. Running is the best hard exercise and stretching is the best soft exercise.

Soft exercise is non-strenuous, easy to do exercise. It is simple and direct, and involves passively stretching your body. It differs from conventional exercise in that it conserves energy instead of using it.

Soft exercise simply involves placing yourself in various positions that allow the outside force of gravity to do all the work for you so that you can stretch all the parts of your body passively. The movements are gymnastic, but they are applied in a way that enables anyone to cultivate, enjoy and experience all the extreme natural movements that the body is capable of making. Soft exercise will act as a natural pain killer, energiser and beautifier. It will stimulate perception, willpower, the quality of orgasm and the joy of life in general. It will help fight heart disease, arthritis, backache as well as slow down the ageing process.

Soft stretching exercises can be done without any equipment, any time anywhere. Stretching brings gymnastics within easy reach of everyone. It is suitable for people of all ages at all levels of fitness from the athlete to the recovering heart patient or ageing arthritic.

Contents

'Don Juan yawned. He lay on his back and stretched his arms and legs. His bones made a cracking sound ...

He stood up, stretching his arms and arching his back like a cat. In spite of his advanced age (he was over seventy years old), his body seemed to be powerful and limber ...

He suggested I should do the same. He said it was a good practice to stretch the entire body after sleeping, sitting or walking ...

"You must stretch your body many times during the day," he said. "The more the better, but only after a long period of work or a long period of rest."'

(Carlos Castaneda
The Teachings of Don Juan)

1. Change Your Life

This book can change your life by introducing you to the simple yet extraordinary world of stretching. A world where it is possible to transform stiffness in any part of your body into suppleness.

No matter how out of shape you may be, how unfit, stiff, tense or old, you can become looser, more relaxed and more energetic than you ever thought possible. With very little preparation and a few elementary instructions anyone who can stand and walk can stretch.

If you are already fit and involved in sport or jogging or dancing, the stretches in this book will make you suppler, more aware and better able to enjoy any activity you do. Even if you are already stretching, practising yoga or gymnastics, this book will take you further.

Whatever your skill you can read about the many benefits of soft exercise and how to make them yours.

In these pages you will learn about the remarkable adaptations the body can make through regular stretching, even in old age. You will learn about stretching

as a natural tranquilliser and energiser
as a posture corrector
as a rejuvenator
as a beautifier
as a pain reliever
as an enhancer of sexual pleasure
as a preparation for pregnancy and childbirth
as a complement to dancing, sports, martial arts, yoga and gymnastics

These claims may strike you as being exaggerated or even ridiculous. You may wonder on what grounds they are based. The full answer to this question will emerge piece by piece, but at this point it is worth explaining how this book came about.

In 1975 a group of ten people agreed to meet for an hour and a half twice weekly. It consisted of two Hatha Yoga teachers, one psychotherapist, one musician, two company directors, one ante-natal teacher, two hair stylists and one housewife. The aim was to find the simplest and most economic means in terms of effort and energy of making their bodies more supple, and to do this by discussing their experiences and exchanging information, difficulties and benefits.

At the beginning of this experiment several members suffered from persistent back pains, migraines, headaches, stiff necks, depressions, sleeplessness, hypertension and fatigue. Over a period of two years these were dramatically improved and in most cases disappeared.

Everyone looked and felt better. Without being self-conscious of posture every member experienced a natural improvement. They also found that the heightened physical awareness that came from stretching ensured that they did not unwillingly misuse and injure their bodies in lifting weights or moving awkwardly. All had gained a first-hand knowledge of their own bodies and found movements generally more enjoyable. One of the women gave birth during these two years and reported that stretching helped her pregnancy, the actual birth and her return to normal. Many felt their love-lives had physically improved. Without exception blood pressures and pulse rates had dropped and breathing had become deeper and lower. These people felt younger and more alive.

The group learned that stretching properly and regularly not only brought suppleness, fitness and more calm, but that it changed emotional and mental functioning. Some remarkable psychological and emotional effects were reported by some members of the group. Cathartic dreams and emotional insights were common experiences. Every member developed a natural self-assurance based on a new-found rootedness in his or her body. They felt emotionally freer, calmer, less anxious and tense and could concentrate better. All were convinced after the end of two years that this type of 'soft exercise' has a healthy effect on the body and a uniquely beneficial effect on the mind.

Before writing this book, the authors, who were members of the group, spent five more years perfecting and teaching others this soft exercise method, again with the same remarkable results.

2. All About Stretching and Stiffness

Life of Movement

Life, the kind we live and see in each other, is made up of what we do. We move, sit, stand, walk, talk, play, work, sing, dance, make love and so on. In all these activities the body, as a whole or part of it, is in motion. And the common indispensable feature is the contraction and relaxation of flesh acting on bones at their joints. These parts form a system, the largest and heaviest body-system known as the body's musculo-skeletal system (Diagrams 1 & 2). This system, directed by the will, is the most prominent and major instrument of everyday life. Regular stretching teaches you to know and understand this instrument. How it or any of its parts functions, its restrictions and possibilities. You learn to care about your body's bony framework, its joints and the powers – muscles, tendons and other soft tissues – that hold it together, support it, position it and move it. Regular stretching is the most basic physical education.

Time for Attention

Most sports are a form of locomotion, you use your entire body to move from place to place through space. The point is to get a result or reach a goal. In tennis it is to hit the ball, in running to cover a particular distance. Your attention is directed outwards, your body taken for granted. The movements involved are complex and rapidly performed so that there is no time to look at the components of movement. Jogging, football, tennis, swimming are all goal-orientated. Stretching, on the other hand, is an analytic tool. It draws your attention to your body's structure, its joints and muscles, how they function and what promotes and restricts their movement. Every stretch gets you to look inwards, you are forced to become aware of your body. There is time enough to analyse, pay attention and care. Stretching is by nature a self-education and analysis as it directs attention inwards to your physical self.

Healing Your Body

Stretching is by its nature a simple technique of paying attention and giving care to your body's system of muscles, bones and joints. But, more important, stretching heals this system, it makes the major instrument of everyday life sound and fit. It does so by gradually making any stiff part of it supple. Regular stretching is an orderly and systematic way of rooting out physical stiffness. It is a musculo-skeletal therapy and education available to practically anyone.

Stiffness

Stiffness is any lack of the natural suppleness or mobility of the limbs and trunk, of their joints and muscles. Obviously stiffness does not mean no movement or mobility at all, it refers to any joint or muscle that is partially stiff; unyielding to some degree. Stiffness describes the loss of full movement natural to joints and muscles.

Stiffness is Universal

Walk down any street and you can see stiff, rigid, tense people everywhere, the older the stiffer. It's like a hidden or neglected epidemic. After heart and lung disorders humanity physically suffers mostly from musculo-skeletal disorders. Backache is nearly as prevalent as the common cold. Most back pain and other musculo-skeletal complaints like arthritis and

3

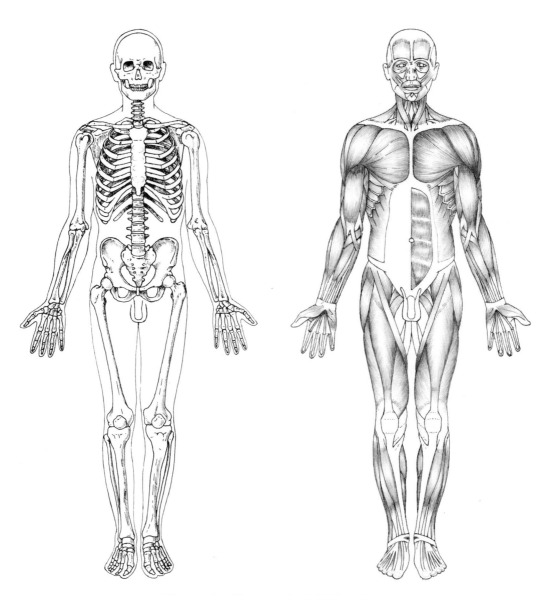

Diagram 1.   The musculo-skeletal system.

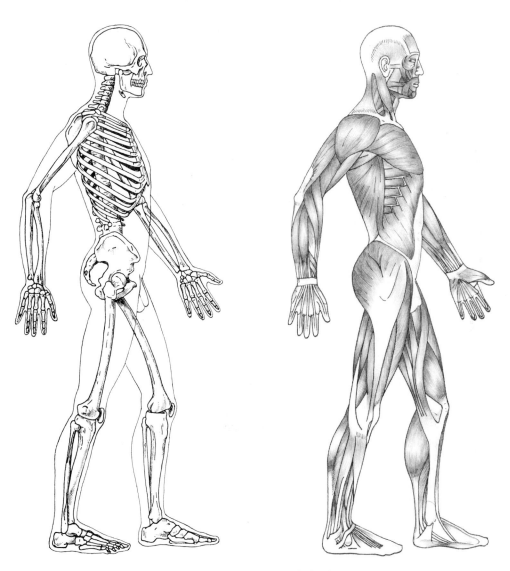

Diagram 2.   The musculo-skeletal system.

rheumatism derive from stiffness. The majority of men and women over fifty, to use an English expression, are 'out of joint'. Stiffness is so common that it is unrecognised and when recognised it is wrongly considered normal and natural, beyond any possibility of repair. The general attitude is that we are stiff because we are made that way, because stiffness is part of getting old and that there is nothing to be done about it.

Stress and Stiffness
Stiffness can be caused by emotional and physical stresses. These are minor traumas from the past that gradually accumulate, and result in physical stiffness. A good example of physical stress can be observed in the experiment of pricking an amoeba. Each time it is pricked and injured it contracts and then expands less, it stiffens. Eventually, pricked enough times it goes totally stiff and rigid, unable to move. An example of emotional stress is the extreme case of fear or threat when one is 'scared stiff' – that is, one's body goes rigid with fear. Because daily life, for the majority of people, demands a small range of movement, the stiffness associated with restricted movement goes unnoticed. Stiffness does not mean no movement or mobility at all. It refers to any joint or muscle that is partially stiff, unyielding to some degree. Stiffness simply describes the loss of full movement that is natural to joints and muscles. Stiffness always restricts movement and distorts posture to some degree (Diagrams 3 & 4).

Stiffness and Pain
The body stiffens naturally to avoid or alleviate pain, both physical and emotional. There are many situations or circumstances that demonstrate this.

We react to a blow to the body by tightening the belly to ward off the blow. When someone is about to receive pain, like taking 'six of the best' on the bottom, the body automatically stiffens and braces up to avoid or lessen the impending pain as much as possible. These are ways by which we defend ourselves against physical pain coming from the outside. Stiffness is also a defence against pain coming from within the body itself. If you dislocate one of your joints to any degree, for whatever reason, the surrounding muscles and tissues stiffen. It is nature's splint to stop you hurting yourself further. Stiffness in this sense is a defensive response against partial dislocation. A stiff neck is dislocated to some degree as its muscles have tightened to hold it together.

If your feelings are hurt in a situation whereby you cannot express, for whatever reasons, strong emotions like crying, fear, anger, and so on, you suppress them by holding your breath, tensing your throat, tightening your belly, lifting and stiffening your shoulders and so on. This way we defend against powerful emotions within us. The body stiffens as a defence against collapsing into infantile emotions like crying, sobbing, screaming, trembling, anger, shouting, and having a tantrum.

The Price of Stiffness
The price we pay is a poorer emotional and motional life. Using the analogy of armour, the price a medieval knight paid for his protection involved the extra weight he had to carry and the restriction, to some degree, of his movements. Now imagine that you put on metal armour made for a knight, and you keep it on indefinitely. What happens to you? Obviously, after a while the weight or load of the armour becomes heavier and begins to be a strain. The weight restricts your movements. They become mechanical, and ungraceful. Your body becomes numb under the load and the strain affects your breathing, your heart, and most of all your muscles and joints that hold you up and move you about. It drains your energy. Eventually, if you keep the armour on long enough you will collapse to the ground fatigued and exhausted. Our criterion or sense of weight is muscle contraction. If you are handed a stone and asked how heavy it is, you will hold it in your hands and say it is not very heavy or heavy or very heavy. You do this by feeling how much your arm muscles have to contract to hold the stone up, the harder they contract the heavier it weighs. A stiff back is a back whose muscles are continually

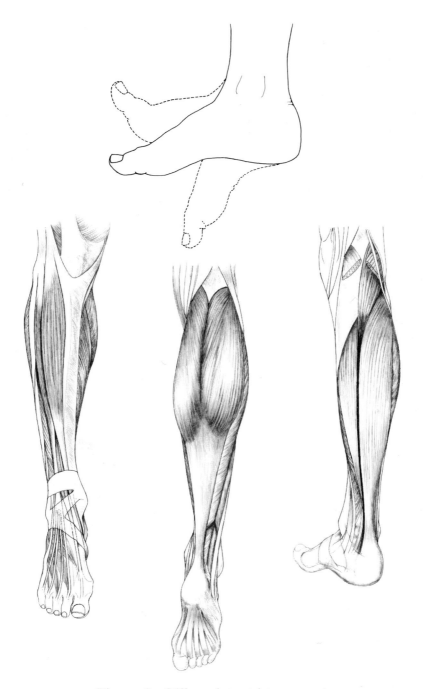

Diagram 3.   Stiff muscles restrict movement.
For example, the foot can make the movements shown in diag. 3a. Pointing the foot straight and bending the foot towards the knee depends on two opposing teams of muscles. Diag. 3b shows the team of muscles that shorten to bend the foot and lengthen to point it. Diags. 3c and 3d show the opposing team of muscles that shorten to point the foot and lengthen to bend it. If these teams cannot fully shorten and lengthen, then the movement of the ankle is partially restricted, the ankle is stiff.

7

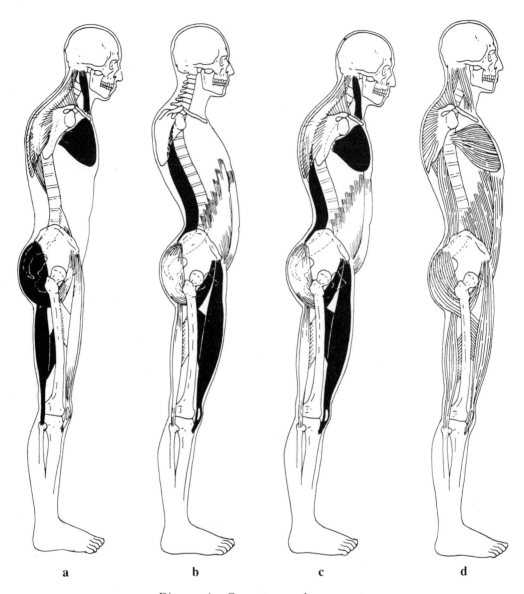

Diagram 4.   On posture and movement.
Muscles work in opposing yet complementary teams. If one team is chronically short its
opposing team is chronically long. Stiff muscle groups distort posture and they can stiffen
at any length. Diag. 4a shows the stiff lengthened muscles (shaded) and the stiff
shortened antagonists (black) associated with round back and round shoulders. Diag. 4b
shows the stiff lengthened muscles (shaded) and the stiff shortened antagonists
associated with hollow back. Diag. 4c shows the stiff lengthened muscles (shaded) and
the stiff shortened muscles (black) associated with rounded back, rounded shoulders and
hollow back. Diag. 4d shows the supple balanced muscles associated with natural
well-balanced posture.

8

in such a state of contraction. It is a back that is holding up an invisible weight, an emotional weight. When you stretch that back it is in a sense like taking off suits of armour from old battles gone by.

Your Choice
Many people including doctors, physiotherapists, osteopaths, and physical trainers don't seem to know that it is possible. Once a person fully realises that with time you can restore suppleness, a choice arises. You can choose to do something positive about any stiffness in your body or choose not to do anything about it and take your chances.

Where It Strikes
It varies in every individual as to which parts of the body get stiff. On the trunk, it can be the neck and throat, the chest and belly, or the back. In the limbs, it can be the hips, knees, ankles, feet, shoulders, wrists, and hands. The body may stiffen virtually everywhere. Some people are slightly stiff everywhere, others have particular stiff areas. Wear and tear, arthritis, happens mostly in the neck, back, hips and knees, and to an extent in the hands and wrists.

Locate Your Stiffness
One could go through life stiff and never be aware of it. Stiffness creeps into one's system gradually and unobtrusively. Often it is not evident to oneself and even less so to others. Aches and pains, tension and tightness are signs that some parts of the body are stiff but these signs are vague. They lack preciseness. Only when you ask your body as a whole or any part of it to go to the limits of its range, does suppleness or stiffness become evident. You have to challenge and test every joint and its relative muscles if you are to know precisely which joints are stiff and how stiff they are. But, because the importance and relevance of stiffness and its opposite suppleness are not common knowledge there is no standard or accepted means of testing suppleness or stiffness. To discover which parts are stiff and the degree of stiffness you would have to place your body in a series of extreme resting positions that expose its suppleness and stiffness. These extreme positions test the major joints, muscles and tendons by taking them to the limits of their range. They are at the same time the means of increasing your suppleness. Cultivating them brings suppleness of your soft tissues and flexibility to your joints and no matter what you do, whether it be playing football, dancing, giving birth or making love, doing it with a supple body improves it. Suppleness is the basic and primary fitness of the body.

The Primary Fitness of the Body
Physical fitness implies a relation between some task to be performed and the individual's physical ability to perform it. It refers to the good condition of the body able to do things like run easily, walk long distances, climb stairs, lift weights and generally be able to do rather strenuous exercise. Suppleness and flexibility are a major part of fitness. Every joint with its relative muscles is designed to perform a series of tasks, that is a series of extreme movements. If they have lost that ability then they are not fit and not in good physical condition. There is a great variety of fitnesses, some related to each other, others not. The fitness of running is basic to all sports that involve running or endurance. But a fit swimmer is not necessarily a fit distance runner and to be fit for weightlifting does not mean a person is also fit for gymnastics or ice skating or cycling.

In the same way that regular jogging makes the body fit for many other strenuous activities like boxing, football, tennis, squash and so on, so regular stretching makes the body fit in terms of suppleness for all activities including running. Regular running and other strenuous activities done with a stiff body may hasten the wear and tear of joints and muscles. It can lead to arthritic and rheumatic disorders depending on the degree of stiffness. In this sense the 'fitness of suppleness' is primary to all other fitnesses. Stretching uses up no energy while running burns up energy. Stretching is the best and most basic soft, passive exercise as running is the best basic hard, active exercise. Regular stretching complements and balances regular jogging and most other sports and activities because it physically relaxes the body.

Relaxation

Stretching is the simplest and most effective way of relaxing your body. It does so by bringing elasticity to the muscles, tendons and other soft tissues that govern the position and movement of your body's bones and joints. Physical relaxation can only be brought about by improving the elasticity of your muscles. Once muscles are stiff they cannot fully relax anymore.

When you lie down and let go of your worries or spend time on a beach or in the countryside without a care in the world you may be superficially relaxed but not necessarily deeply relaxed as your very fibres and tissues could be tense and tight. The reason is that there are two kinds of tension. First of all there is the kind of muscle tension which results from a here and now mental or physical stressful situation. This is simply the action of muscles in particular circumstances. This kind of tension eases as soon as a stressful situation eases. But the kind of tension we are talking about is radically different. It is the kind of tension that is inherent in the muscle tissue itself. It is the result of all the unresolved situations of the past, all the strains, physical and mental, the wear and tear of life. This wear and tear builds up in the tissues. They stiffen defensively and lose their natural elasticity.

You can never stop muscle-tensing situations from arising but you can lessen the deep tension that has built up over time. Muscles register stress. If the slate is not wiped clean regularly these registrations accumulate, stiffness develops, and your ability to relax physically is lessened. Your body has the remarkable property of adaption. As it can adapt to temperature change, drastic changes in food intake, cigarette smoking, and pollution, so it adapts to accumulative tension and stiffness. It cuts off the sensation of stiffness and actually becomes numb to it. Adaption is essential if the body is to function comfortably under specific conditions but it is not necessarily good for you. Because your body may adapt to very cold or very hot temperatures, to minimum or excessive food intake, to sixty cigarettes a day, to diesel and petrol fumes, it does not mean that these things are O.K. For short periods, maybe, but for long periods you take your chances. You can get away with stiffness for short periods of time but over and above that you run the risk of back pain, arthritis, high blood pressure, and heart and other problems that can be associated with excessive tension and the inability to relax fully.

3. The Impact of Stretching

The Impact on Your Breathing

Your lungs play a passive role in breathing; expanding when your chest enlarges and recoiling when it reduces in size. So, breathing mechanically depends on the opening and closing of your chest. The muscles primarily responsible for this action are your diaphragm at the bottom of your chest which enlarges your chest from top to bottom and your intercostals between the ribs which enlarge your chest both from side to side and from back to front. These primary breathing muscles are closely associated with neighbouring muscles which in turn are associated with the rest of your body's muscles. So that every breath you breathe depends on the co-ordinated activity of many muscles.

Your head, neck and shoulder muscles influence your intercostals, and your abdominal and pelvic muscles influence your diaphragm. The muscles of your spinal column have an effect on both those primary breathing muscles. The top part of the spine directly supports your chest and intercostals and the bottom part is attached and anchored to your diaphragm.

If your diaphragm and intercostals are stiff and inelastic it is obvious that your breathing will be directly restricted. But any stiffness in the neighbouring muscles will also restrict, to some extent, the opening and closing of your chest in breathing. Check this out for yourself.

Tilt your pelvis down as far as possible with your buttocks lifted up and notice the restricting effect it has on your breathing. Now breathe with your pelvis in the reverse position, that is pulled up with your abdominal muscles tight and pulled in, and notice a similar effect. Now try rounding your shoulders and holding your chest in while breathing or holding it expanded and rigid and notice the restrictions on your breathing.

The most important muscles in breathing besides your intercostals and diaphragm are those of your abdomen or belly. These act in direct harmony with your diaphragm. As your diaphragm contracts your abdominal muscles relax and as your diaphragm relaxes your abdominal muscles contract.

As you breathe in your diaphragm moves down to make your chest cavity longer. As it moves down it presses upon your abdominal organs which in turn push your belly wall forward. Now if your abdominal muscles are stiff and tense they resist the downward pull of your diaphragm and your chest cavity cannot lengthen fully. This restricts deep breathing. So there is no doubt that tight, inelastic abdominal muscles directly hamper the actions of your diaphragm, and therefore the depth of your breathing movement.

Stretching your body, especially areas like your abdomen, back, shoulders, neck and hips, over time will improve your breathing.

Your spine actually moves (or should move) when you breathe. It straightens slightly when you breathe in and collapses when you breathe out. Your back is an integral part of your breathing mechanism and the more you rotate it, bend it backwards, sideways, forwards, the more flexible it will be and more positive an influence it will have on your chest, on your breathing movements and on your breathing as a whole.

Stretching your neck is important to your breathing. First because it centres the position of your head. If your head is held off centre (and it is in many people), it throws a strain on your spine and chest which affects your breathing capacity. Also all the large muscles of your neck are attached to the top of your chest or spine in some way. The less stiffness in these muscles, the less they will restrict your chest and your breathing.

All the muscles of your shoulders directly or indirectly associate with those of your neck, chest and spine. The freer your shoulders are the freer your neck and back and the less cramped your chest will be and the freer your breathing. So, stretching your shoulders improves your breathing.

Stretching your hips improves your breathing as the large muscles of your hips are closely associated with your abdominal and lower back muscles. We have already mentioned the importance of the abdominal muscles while the lower back muscles are important because they in turn relate to the rest of your spine.

Consistent stretching increases the capacity of your chest and thus your lungs' volume of air. This can be easily measured by a breathometer which measures the volume of air of a maximum inhalation and exhalation. The rate of breathing in a resting position (breaths per minute) before and after a stretch session can also be measured and is immediately a bit lower. This rate is significantly lowered after several years of regular stretching. Every stiff inelastic muscle indirectly involved in the action of breathing which is made supple through stretching contributes to some extent to a freer, deeper, more relaxed breathing movement.

The Impact on Your Circulation

When muscles are stiff, blood cannot permeate all the tissue and will seek alternative routes. This can in time render a muscle even stiffer by drying it out and causing a build-up of waste products. This often happens in old age. A muscle that is regularly stretched, that keeps its elastic quality, allows blood to flow through it freely and is able to receive all the nourishment it needs to keep it healthy. Furthermore, fully elastic muscles enable blood to carry away their waste products more effectively. Stiff muscles become clogged with toxic waste, they become polluted. Elasticity, nourishment and removal of wastes go hand in hand.

There are three forces that drive blood around your body: your heart, your breathing movements and the muscle action of your legs and feet. Your heart has enough power to send blood to all the tissues but does not provide enough force to return it. It needs assistance. This is where relaxed and deep breathing movements are a great asset. Alternating negative and positive pressures in your chest and abdominal cavities caused by breathing both sucks and pushes blood up through your trunk. Stretching all the muscles that are indirectly and directly active in breathing not only improves the quality of your breathing as seen in the last section, but also indirectly assists your circulation. As for your leg muscles, all their contractions when you are walking, standing or moving around, have a pumping effect on the veins that run between and over them. This squeezes blood upwards towards your heart. So your heart to a large extent depends upon your skeletal muscles for assistance in circulating your blood. It is helped indirectly by your breathing muscles and directly by your leg muscles. Stretching gives your muscles the elasticity they need to be able to help pump blood back to your heart as efficiently as possible.

Everyone knows that blood delivers nutrients (especially oxygen) to all the cells of the body and that it removes waste. Less well known is the fact that all cells are bathed in a defensive fluid called lymph. Lymph fights off invading bacteria and viruses and like blood it circulates around your body. It is manufactured in various glands throughout your body. Lymph relies mostly on the compression of muscles and the suction and pressure of your breathing movements for its circulation. Obviously the freer your lymph flow the better is your body's defence against bacteria and viruses. Stretching your body regularly, and so improving the action of your muscles and the quality of your breathing movements, keeps your lymph moving more freely.

The Impact on Your Perception

Many people are self-conscious about their body instead of being aware of their body. They are stuck with a picture, image or concept of their body in their mind. Authentic body-awareness, however, involves no thinking at all. It is the direct internal perception of your physical self. This body perception or awareness is your most basic sense.

As the eyes can be compared to a camera and the ears to a microphone, in the same way every physical receptor can be compared to a carpenter's spirit-level. In your inner ears, muscles, tendons and joints are a complex network of tiny spirit-levels giving you your sense of spatial magnitude, weight, balance, position, and movement.

When your muscles, tendons and joints are stiff these physical receptors are dulled and partially numbed, when supple they are sharp. So that every stiff, inelastic muscle group made supple through stretching adds to some extent to the keenness of your sense of your physical self. There are very few activities that heighten muscle sensitivity as effectively as consistent stretching.

The Impact on Your Will
The will is a force, a power, a kind of control from within. It is a link or relation between ourselves and the world. Now stop reading for a few moments. Get up from your sitting position. Lie on the floor for a few seconds and return to sitting and reading. Do this before reading on. If you ask yourself how you did this, you will realise that you merely willed yourself to stop reading, lie down and return to reading. You just did it. You made the decision and went ahead. You did not concern yourself whether muscles were contracting or stretching, which part to move first and so on. You just willed it and it all happened. Postures and movements of your body are voluntary, whether you are aware of it or not. To move or position your body or any part of it involves the decision to do so, the exercise of your will.

The link between will and brain-muscle action is a mystery. It is not known how the decision to move triggers off the appropriate brain activity that results in the desired action. Immanuel Kant said, 'That my will moves my arm is to me no more comprehensible than if someone should say that it could hold back the moon itself'. So we see that there are two aspects of every conscious action. One is the mechanical action of muscles, bones, joints and so on controlled by the nervous system and the brain. The other is the inner decision and judgment, the will. This continual play of muscle action and will is mostly unconscious. No amount of willing, however, can get your body to adopt positions or make movements that take it to the naturally designed limits of its range unless your body is supple enough. Your will depends upon the co-operation of your body's muscles and nervous system.

So the more efficient the action of your muscles, the more effective the operation of your will, and the more command you will have over your body.

Carlos Castaneda, who spent several years with a Yaqui Indian together as teacher and pupil, writes this:

Don Juan laughed and patted my chest and made a joke about a Mexican weightlifter who had enormous pectoral muscles but could not do heavy physical labour because his back was weak. 'Watch those muscles,' he said. 'They shouldn't be just for show.'

'My muscles have nothing to do with what you're talking about,' I said in a belligerent mood. 'They do,' he replied. 'The body must be perfection (i.e. totally perfectly supple and fit) before the will is a functioning unit...' Perhaps the first thing one should do is to know that one can develop the will.

Stretching the muscles that govern joints improves the possible brain activity and muscle action at those joints, and indirectly influences and improves the operation of the will.

The Impact on Your Beauty
Beauty is that combination of qualities which gives keen pleasure to your senses, especially that of sight. Beauty is not only skin deep – it is also structural. Besides the weight, the figure, shape and posture of your body are determined by the size and shape of your bones and by their relationship to one another at their joints. The size and shape of your bones themselves cannot be changed, but their relationship can. By increasing the flexibility of your joints you

automatically improve the positioning of your body when standing, sitting, walking and so on, in everyday upright positions.

Whether you are short, tall, or of medium build, stretching can improve your figure. The most profound change can be in the area of the neck, shoulders and chest, making a vast difference to your build within the limits of the physique you were born with. Stretching over time can improve the positioning of your head and neck; change rounded shoulders into well-balanced shoulders; open the chest; reduce the protrusion of your belly; improve the position of your pelvis (tucking in your buttocks); dramatically decrease the curves of your spinal column, and so on. These changes all increase the beauty of your body.

Besides changing your bodily frame, stretching will also improve the shape, definition and tone of the muscles themselves. By improving their function their form naturally improves. For example, the shape of your legs (calves, thighs and buttocks) changes noticeably for the better when your hip, knee and ankle joints are more flexible and the muscles governing them more elastic, supple and relaxable.

Graceful movement is simply a natural ease of movement. It is something that happens naturally to you when you start stretching regularly, when your body becomes more relaxed and your structure gradually starts to change. You don't have to think about it or become self-conscious of it. Grace is a by-product of stretching.

Stretching over time increases the overall relaxation of your body. This is reflected in the eyes, they become softer and brighter, and in the expression of the facial muscles, they become less tense and strained, and the more relaxed your face becomes through stretching the more beautiful it will be.

Another contribution to beauty is the condition of the skin. Because stretching over time improves blood and lymph circulation, it also improves the colour and tone of the skin.

So altogether every stiff muscle made supple through stretching will add to some degree to increasing the beauty of your figure, your face, your skin and your movements.

The Impact on Your Energy

Consistent stretching reduces fatigue and heaviness and brings an overall feeling of bodily lightness and energy. And to feel light and energetic is undoubtedly one of the greatest physical experiences.

Lightness is an experience (or quality) of little weight, pressure or force. Heaviness, its opposite, is an experience of great weight, pressure or force. Your experience of lightness and weight is actually determined by your muscle sense (proprioception). It is determined by the degree and amount of muscles contracting. The greater the contraction the greater the experience of weight. Lift a heavy weight like a table or a piano and you will experience its weight through the contraction and resistance of your muscles. Hold it up long enough and you will fatigue. Muscles can also contract without any apparent weight. For example contract your fist, elbow and shoulder, squeeze hard, you are not gripping and lifting an outside weight yet the experience is the same as if you were. Hold the squeeze long enough and in time you will also fatigue.

From these two simple examples it is obvious that when muscles contract sufficiently energy is used up and you experience tightness, tension or weight. And when muscles are stiff or inelastic, they are contracting, using up energy and bringing on the feeling of heaviness. This loss of energy and feeling of heaviness from stiff muscles is accumulative.

As continual stretching increases elasticity it increases one's feelings of lightness and energy, energy being the capacity for action, for doing things. Indeed, every stiff inelastic muscle that is made supple through stretching contributes to some degree to feeling light and more energetic.

The Impact on Your Muscular Armour

The expression 'bodily armour' was introduced by Wilhelm Reich. He claimed that behind every group of stiff, tense muscles there existed a blocked feeling or emotion; that body armour was a protective manoeuvre against catastrophic situations, trauma and pain. He tried to find a series of exercises that could dissolve physical stiffness methodically. He failed as he used muscle-building and resisting exercises. After much trial and error his final method of releasing these blocks and opening up the body and mind was to provoke the blocked feeling or emotion which governed the particular defensive muscle actions. Because emotional defences governed muscular defences, Reich assumed that the only way to break down physical armour was through the emotional armour behind it, and not vice versa; that freeing the physical defences could not open up and free the emotional ones. On the other hand the 'Alexander Technique' and 'Rolfing' both claim to break down the emotional blocks through loosening up physical armour.

Consistent stretching gradually loosens up the stiff muscles that make up bodily armour. This is a slow but sure process that gently dismantles the blocked emotions behind the armour. These released emotions are expressed in dreams and in everyday situations. One becomes less defensive physically and emotionally.

If Reich had come across the technique of stretching when he was looking for a physical way to break down muscular armour he would probably have cultivated and used it.

The Impact on Your Sex Life
Regular stretching changes your sex life in several ways. Not only does it enable you to use a greater variety of love positions, but also, more importantly, it will physically improve the quality of your orgasms.

Every time we make love it involves a combination (or series of combinations) of two individual bodily positions. The more supple your body and your partner's body (especially the pelvis, lower back, thighs, knees and ankles) the greater is the variety of love positions possible. And most evidence, ancient and modern, suggests that using a variety of love positions increases the range of pleasures and adds spice to one's love-making.

Orgasm is an experience that is not open to outside evaluation. Only you know whether the quality of your experience is full or partial, satisfying or unsatisfying. Yet sex is a physical function that depends upon the suppleness, vitality and awareness of your body for its pleasure and satisfaction. Unsatisfactory or partial orgasm is often bound to physical disturbances in the form of fatigue, lack of body awareness, restricted movement and lack of suppleness especially in the trunk, pelvis and legs.

Most of us fail to appreciate the importance of movement in orgastic experiences. We think mostly about the contact part of love-making to the neglect of the movement part. Generally, we mistakenly assume that sexual movements serve only to increase the friction between genital organs. Kinesthetic pleasure (the pleasure derived from sexual movements) depends on the quality of your pelvic and spinal movements. The freer and fuller these movements of the pelvis and trunk the greater the pleasure. Stiffness limits sexual movements and motion and reduces kinesthetic pleasure and hence the quality of your orgasms.

Many people are unaware of the low energetic state of their bodies. Yet one's sexual response depends heavily upon the availability of excess energy. Stiffness involves the constant presence of bound-up, undischarged muscular energy, while suppleness is free of this so that the energy that otherwise would be used in keeping muscles in some kind of contraction, is then available for other bodily activities, like orgasm.

Conditions of fatigue, over-tiredness or exhaustion greatly diminish sexual feelings and orgasms. By contrast, the fitter, suppler and more energetic person has a greater chance of a stronger, more complete sexual response. Your body is the one and only instrument of your sexual feelings and it is your direct perception or awareness of it, together with suppleness and vitality, that determines to a large extent the quality of your orgasms. The soft stretching exercises of chapters 6 and 7 – when cultivated – will result in suppleness, vitality and body-awareness. Stretching regularly will help you to get back in shape, to 'tune the instrument', to get physically the most out of your sex life.

The Impact on Your Health

The most common physical disorders are heart troubles, breathing disorders and disorders of the joints and muscles. As stretching improves circulation, by lowering your pulse rate, blood pressure and blood temperature, it contributes to alleviating and preventing disorders of the heart. As stretching increases the capacity of your chest and the efficiency of your principal breathing muscles it contributes to alleviating and preventing breathing disorders. As stretching improves the functioning and flexibility of joints and the elasticity and relaxability of muscles it contributes to alleviating and preventing disorders of the joints and muscles. And back pains, headaches, arthritis and rheumatic pains are all disorders of the musculo-skeletal system.

The Impact on Your Ageing

Gradual stiffness is part of the process of ageing. No one can stop the process of ageing. Through constant stretching, however, one can slow it down considerably.

If you start stretching your body regularly when you are young you can maintain its elasticity. If you start a little older you can eventually regain any lost elasticity and then maintain what you have regained. If you start late in life you will probably never fully regain the suppleness of youth but you will definitely slow down the stiffening process. All the benefits of stretching, that is, improved flexibility, elasticity, relaxation, breathing, circulation, physical perception, will, beauty, energy, and lightness, will add up and contribute to 'youth'. This is probably the most attractive result of stretching consistently over the years and is the result most highly appreciated and remarked on by those that have practised stretching for some time.

4. Feel Your Own Anatomy

When you stretch regularly you learn about your own body. There is a vast difference between studying anatomy or directly perceiving your own personal anatomy through your muscle sense. Academic anatomy artificially divides the body into parts to discover their position, structure and function. You learn about it through the use of your mind's eye, through visualisation. One can be a lecturer in the subject and yet have very little sense of one's own personal anatomy. On the other hand, one can be a skilled gymnast having great intuitive knowledge of one's own body yet be totally ignorant of any scientific anatomy.

Stretching draws your attention to the parts of your body that are at the limits of their range. It's an analytic tool and results in the natural division of your body by your muscle sense in the here and now.

Through regular stretching you experience the location of your joints (and there is quite a difference between knowing where, for example, your knees are or experiencing your knees), and you learn the present and potential range of the joints you exercise. You learn the overall feeling of your body's structure. You experience the location of the soft parts (muscles, tendons) that govern your joints and their degree of elasticity. The series of exercises presented in this book are directed at the major joints of the body, and their soft parts, those of the spinal column, hips, knees, ankles, feet, shoulders, elbows, wrists and hands. By cultivating these stretches you improve your direct perception of all these parts, automatically without having to visualise or think about them.

Feel Your Muscle Action

Just sitting and reading this book depends on a series of opposing muscle contractions and stretchings. When you swallow, fidget, move your arms and legs or just sit upright, no matter what, muscles are contracting and relaxing to make this possible.

Each joint is moved by two opposing teams of muscles – the flexors and extensors. Their action is simply demonstrated by bending your elbow or knee (Diagram 5).

When you straighten your knee the extensors shorten behind and the flexors stretch in front. When you bend your knee the flexors shorten and the extensors stretch. It's like a tug-of-war, one team can gain only what the other loses. In short, muscles work joints in opposing yet complementary paired teams. When one team is fully shortening the other is fully stretching.

To find out in your own body which muscles are active and which are antagonistically passive in any movement at any joint, simply resist the movement. The active muscle group will contract forcefully and the passive group will go limp. For example, bend your elbow and resist the movement. Your biceps and its assisting muscles will tighten and the opposing group of muscles, your triceps, will go limp (See diagram 6a). If you now try and straighten your elbow and resist the movement, the reverse happens. Your triceps will harden and your biceps will soften. This resistance of movement can be used at any freely movable joint in your body – your hips, knees, ankles, elbows, wrists and so on. With this technique one can find the flexors, extensors, abductors, adductors, and the inward and outward rotators at any and every joint. One need never refer to an anatomy book to find out which of one's muscles are active or passive in any given movement. Whenever you want to define which muscle groups are being stretched in a stretching exercise, just make the opposite movement and resist it. The muscles that harden and increase in definition are those being stretched.

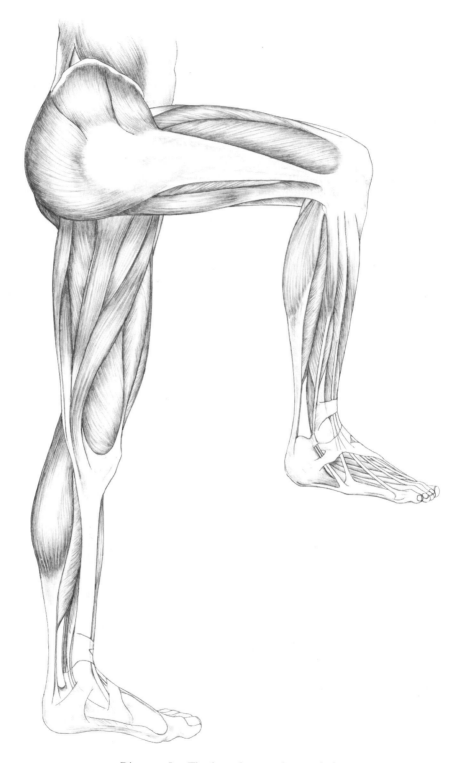

Diagram 5.   The knee bent and extended.

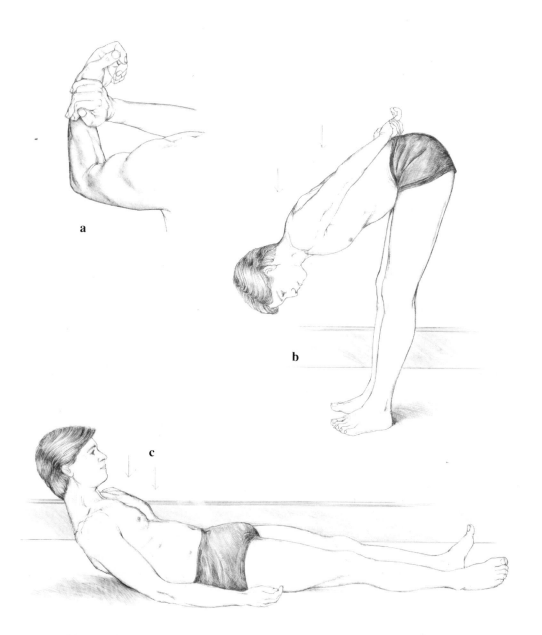

Diagram 6.   a. Resisted movement.   b. Assisted by gravity.   c. Resisting gravity.

Feel the Force of Gravity

A vital fact is that all movements of bones at their joints are either resisted or assisted by gravity. If you lie on your back and lift your head and trunk a little for a few seconds, the force of gravity resists the movement and you will sense your neck and abdominal muscles tightening to shorten and pull your head and trunk upwards (See diagram 6c). The moment any part of your body meets enough resistance, muscle contraction takes place and is experienced as tightening or tension. If you stand up with legs slightly apart, and bend forward towards your toes with back and knees straight, gravity assists the movement with no tightening of your neck and abdominal muscles (See diagram 6b). You will then sense your back thigh muscles, especially behind your knees, stretching, perhaps even painfully. When the range of movement or position of your body or any part of it is extreme enough, and assisted by gravity or any other force, muscle relaxation takes place and is experienced as stretching. In every stretch try to sense the force of gravity and know which muscle groups are assisted by gravity and which are resisted by gravity.

Feel and Stretch Your Body with Your Own Hands

Each one of us in endowed with a unique body. However, one could go through life without ever having given full attention to this gift through one's own intimate touch. Massaging our bodies instinctively and intuitively is a fundamental way of experiencing our anatomy. Practised regularly and methodically like stretching, self-massage improves the condition, feeling and sense of one's own body. Stretching and self-massage have much in common. Both release hidden tensions and pains, stimulate blood and lymph flow, give elasticity to muscle-tendon tissue and bring awareness to those areas worked on. Massage is a form of stretching. Heat and pressure from the fingers not only stimulates blood flow, disperses hidden tensions and pains and softens muscles and tendons, but also directly prepares the soft tissues of the body for stretching exercises.

There is no mystery in massage but those who try it are surprised at the power they hold in their hands. Rubbing a painful part of the body is instinctive, natural and soothing. Massage is one of the most ancient methods of healing and has been used in different forms for many thousands of years. The advantage of self-massage over being massaged by another person is that you learn about your body through your own hands. Another person will be able to get to some parts more easily than you can and the technique used may be more professional and efficient. Yet you can with curiosity, practice and patience, learn to reach all parts of your body and develop your own natural techniques. You will discover how to do this instinctively and will have the advantage of regulating the pressure to suit yourself. Massage, especially deep massage, provokes pain. The reaction varies in different people and in different parts of the body. Your body may be full of painful spots you are never aware of until you try massage. Mongolian warriors equated unnecessary painful spots with fear and before and after battle they would massage their entire bodies to rid themselves of pain, and hence hidden fear.

Self-massage enables you to separate the soft from the hard tissues of your body. Soft tissue can get gummed up or stuck to bone where it should be free to glide smoothly. One learns how to glean the soft muscle-tendon tissue from the bones it runs alongside and is attached to. It is quite easy to massage painful spots away. All you need do is explore, press and probe to find the painful parts and then use your fingers and thumbs to rub them away and dissolve the pain.

Develop your own system of massage that will allow you to get thoroughly acquainted with your body. You can take a different area each week. Begin with your hands, find all the tender parts and gradually dissolve them. Then try your feet. Feet are common sites for mechanical strain and chemical waste and may be extremely tender in some parts. Then work up from your ankles to your knees, and then your groin and abdomen and so on. Self-massage can be done whenever you set aside the time. Ten or fifteen minutes before going to bed or upon rising seems to be the easiest time for some people. For other people in the bath or any other leisure time is more suitable. A half hour on your hands alone each day for one month (fifteen hours) will convey the whole point of intuitive massage and give immense benefit. No one can teach you how to 'handle' your own body. No one can do it for you as well as you if you have the discipline to develop your own skills.

Massage in itself is a form of stretching, it is manual stretching, and as such it is an ideal complement to stretching exercise. An ideal time to use it is before a stretch session. Soft tissue stretches/lengthens more easily when it has been massaged beforehand. If you have a particularly stiff area, one calf for example may be stiffer than the other, you may prepare the calf muscles for the appropriate stretching exercises by working them with your hands for five minutes. You will be surprised at the reduction in resistance when you stretch.

As stretching is the ideal complement to all activity and sport so is massage an ideal complement to stretching. Whether you are stretching for the sake of stretching itself or use it to improve your chosen activity or sport, intuitive self-massage will enable you to stretch more easily and freely, and in its own right is a perfect body conditioner.

5. The Art of Stretching

Anyone can, and everyone is, capable of stretching. You need no specific physical skill or ability to stretch. Whatever your age, however stiff or supple you are, you can get the best from stretching to suit your own body.

The very nature of soft stretching makes it perfectly safe. Most of the stretches allow you to go to your full range of movements with your body in a well supported or resting position. If you do have any kind of ailment or injury, it is advisable to tell your doctor, osteopath, or whoever is treating you that you are planning to stretch. He can tell you whether or not your condition may be aggravated by stretching.

No Contest

Each person's body is unique and each will vary at the start in their range of movement. Some will be stiffer or looser than others in particular stretches. This is unimportant! Whether you stretch alone, in twos, or in a group, there is no contest. Go as slowly as you need to for your own comfort. Everyone differs in their flexibility and elasticity, the important thing, the thing we all have in common, is that we are all capable of stretching our bodies. Carry out your own stretches gradually, the emphasis should be on the feel of the stretch not on how far you can stretch, that will come later. There is no instant way to relax the body. You will discover that natural improvement, at your own pace, will give you the most pleasure.

Anytime, Anywhere

You can stretch whenever you feel like it. You may feel like a daily half hour session alone and undisturbed or you can use specific stretches that can be done almost anywhere, anytime. You can stretch at work, on the beach, in the lift, while walking, in a field, after sitting, standing or driving for long periods, or before and after sleeping or resting. You can stretch while watching TV, all the sitting stretches are ideal and at the end of a film or show you will have given your hips, knees and ankles a complete work-out. Stopping at traffic lights is an ideal opportunity to stretch your neck. When your body and mind feel tense and you feel too irritable to stretch it may be the best time to do so. A highlight of stretching is the way in which it deals with the kind of tension initiated by irritability.

Once you slip into the subtleties of stretching you will see that it is possible to stretch some part of your body at almost any place any time.

Keep Breathing

The point to remember while stretching is neither to hold your breath nor over breathe. Stretching gets the best results when you breathe normally and smoothly. Do not make a feature out of breathing, just remember to keep breathing. Try to breathe through your nose as it is more physically relaxing. If you feel like going beyond your limit from time to time as one does with stretching, inhaling and exhaling smoothly and consciously makes it easier. However, sometimes the pain of overstretching may cause you to gasp or blow. Overstretching is not recommended but if you do experience difficulty in breathing at the height of a stretch, try to control your breathing through your throat. Purposefully inhale and exhale from your throat. As your body adapts to stretching so will your breathing patterns and rhythms.

22

Time Tells

There is no essential set time to spend in any stretch. Please yourself and let your own sensations guide you. However, based on our experience we have suggested timings for each stretch, but these are only rough guides. Some are better as long stretches, while others are more effective as quick stretches. Yet thirty seconds in a stretch will be more beneficial than ten seconds. If you have forty-five minutes free you can take nine of the basic resting stretches and spend five minutes in each one. If you have ten minutes you can cover the whole body with a stretch a minute. So you can vary stretching to suit your needs and circumstances at any given time. Ideally, the stiff beginner should start with the shorter timings and grow into the longer ones. But only you will know when you have had enough.

The Potency of Gravity

One of the remarkable things about soft stretching is the way it harnesses the outside force of gravity and uses it for its own ends. With soft exercise you don't fight or resist gravity, you surrender to it. This has an extraordinary effect on your energy. You not only get energy from the stretches themselves, but you also save energy in the process of doing them. This gives gravity assisted stretching its immense potency. So remember through all the stretches: let go and allow the gravitational pull of your body to work for you.

Play With It

Once you become familiar with the stretches you can play with them. There are many nuances and variations of all the stretches. You may find yourself changing the angle, direction and momentum in many of them. Here stretching ceases to become just an exercise and becomes an intuitive activity.

Good Sides and Bad Sides

In some of the stretches you will discover that you have a good side and a bad side. In other words one shoulder, knee or leg may be stiffer than its opposite. Most people experience this at some time to some extent. Give the stiffer side the careful and gradual attention it needs until it catches up with the good side. In this way stretching effectively balances out your body. Many people have an unconscious tendency to shy away from their stiffer areas. However, balancing out the stiffer areas with looser ones will accelerate your progress in cultivating overall suppleness and flexibility.

Free to Move

The less clothing you wear during stretching the better. Whatever you choose should be loose and comfortable. At home bare feet are recommended. Outdoors or in a studio or gym any kind of soft shoe will do.

Feel Your Way

To get the best from your stretches, stretch within your limits without straining. Going too far too quickly may be painful and over stretching may leave you with sore muscles for some time after. On the other hand, if you stretch too easily and timidly you will find it boring and ineffective. There is a stretch lying between these two extremes. A stretch that becomes effortless and increasingly potent with regular practice, a stretch that will reveal itself to you without difficulty. You will learn to stretch by how you feel, by using the sensations that come from your body as a guide. Take the stretch far enough to feel it. It always helps to concentrate on the stretch. This enables your muscles to relax and let go more readily. When you feel the stretch become easier then you can take it a little further.

6. Soft Exercises: stretches 1 – 57

1. Sit on your heels facing a wall about an arm's length away and spread your knees comfortably apart. Raise your arms with elbows straight, lean your body forward and place your hands on the wall shoulder width apart. When on the wall make sure your elbows are locked straight and your fingers and palms extended to their limits. Then lift your chest forward to the wall and at the same time draw your shoulder-blades together and down at the back (chest and breast bone lifting, shoulder-blades dropping). Breathe smoothly and feel the stretch. Try half a minute at first and eventually build up to several minutes. Feel the stretch in your shoulders and arms.

2. Lie on your back with your buttocks as close to a wall as possible. Place your feet on the wall so that your knees come close to your chest. Raise your arms shoulder width apart with elbows straight and slowly take them over your head onto the floor behind you. As you do this draw your shoulder-blades down towards your lower back. This stretch is only effective when you keep your shoulder-blades tightly drawn down your back. Make sure you do not arch your back or lift your chest to make the movement. Try one minute for a short stretch and then build up to three and then five minutes for a longer stretch.

3. Sitting on the floor put your hands out behind you, palms down, keep your hands at shoulder width. Edge your buttocks and legs forward, keeping your hands in the same position until you feel the stretch in the front of your shoulders. Keep your shoulders down and away from your head and ears. Quick stretch thirty seconds, long stretch one to several minutes. Reverse your palms (face up) and repeat. Remember to keep your hands at shoulder width and your shoulders drawn downwards away from your head.

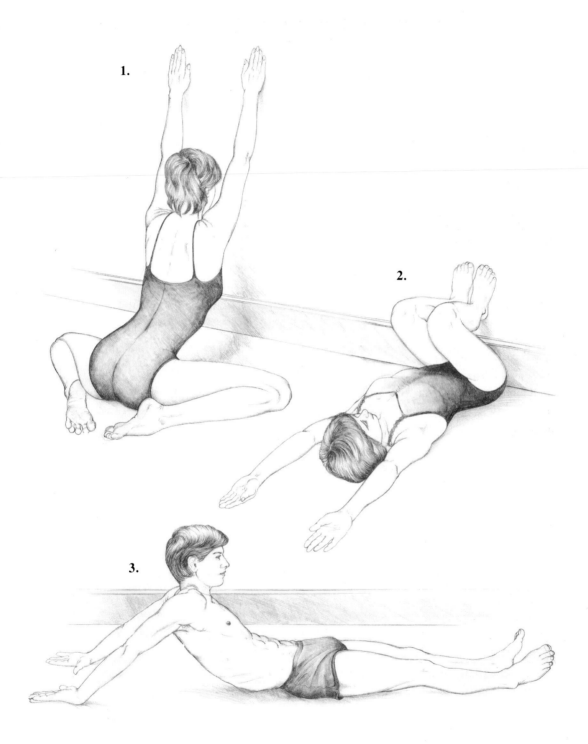

1.

2.

3.

25

4a. Drop your head slightly forward, bring one arm up behind it and slightly bend your elbow. Pull on the elbow with your other hand. Stretch gradually. Ten to fifteen seconds.

4b. Change your line of pull to downwards and increase the stretch bending the elbow into a V shape. Ten to fifteen seconds.

5. Place your palms together behind your back, fingers pointing downwards. Then rotate your wrists so that your fingers are pointing up your back. Draw your elbows back, your shoulder-blades downwards and press the heels of your palms towards each other. Thirty seconds for a short stretch and one to several minutes for a long stretch.

6. Take one arm behind your back and bend slightly. With your other hand pull your elbow across the mid-line of your back. Try half a minute and repeat other side.

7. Place one arm as far up your back as possible as if to touch your head. Stretch the other arm up and overhead and link your fingers behind your back. When linked take the top elbow backwards and downwards and the bottom elbow backwards and upwards. If this is easy stay in it for thirty seconds then reverse arms and repeat other side. If you cannot link your fingers together use a towel or belt to assist you.

8a. Arms at shoulder height in front of you, palms facing each other. Keeping your arms at that level slowly take them backwards making sure that you extend your fingers and palms to their limits and use only your arms and shoulders to make the movement. As you take your arms back do not involve your head and neck in the movement. Keep your head and trunk steady and let your shoulders do all the work. This stretch is not effective if you lean forward or lift your shoulders. Fifteen seconds is ample for the stretch. Repeat several times.

8b. A a variation of this stand in a doorway. Grab the frame at shoulder height and edge forward through the doorway until your arms are at full stretch. Slowly walk forwards until your legs and trunk are vertical. Quick stretch fifteen seconds, long stretch thirty seconds.

N.B. With all these shoulder stretches you may feel it in the armpits, at the back of the shoulder or at the top of your arms. The sensations differ in the various areas. Eventually the kinks iron out and you get a smooth overall stretch.

26

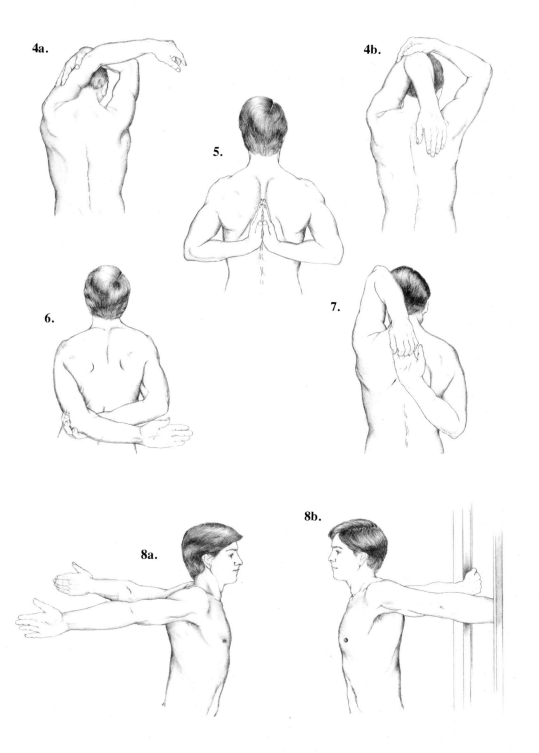

4a.

4b.

5.

6.

7.

8a.

8b.

27

9. Lie on your front with your hands in front of you. Come up onto your elbows with your wrists together and cup your hands under your chin. Make sure your elbows are well forward and a few inches apart. Keep your shoulders and shoulder-blades downwards away from your chin. Now gently take your head back as far as possible stretching and lifting your throat and upper chest. At the same time draw your shoulders and upper back downwards towards your lower back. The point is to lift your front off the floor and drop your upper back and shoulders down towards the floor. This stretch is only effective if the tips of your shoulders are kept at maximum distance from your ears. Half a minute to a minute.

10. From lying on your front come up onto your elbows. Your elbows should be not more than shoulder width apart and your upper arms vertical. Tighten your buttocks and drop your shoulders down towards your lower back, pressing your lower back forward towards the floor. At the same time lift and stretch the front of your body from your navel to the top of your chest. Hold for fifteen seconds to half a minute.

11. In the same position as exercise ten lift one leg and place your foot on the floor on the side of your other leg about twelve inches from it. Keep both your elbows on the floor and your buttocks tight. Stay in it for five seconds and then repeat with the other leg. Repeat several times alternating legs for a minute or so. Remember to keep breathing smoothly and evenly throughout all the stretches.

9.

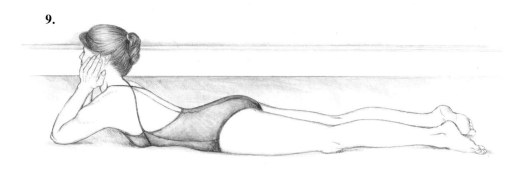

10.

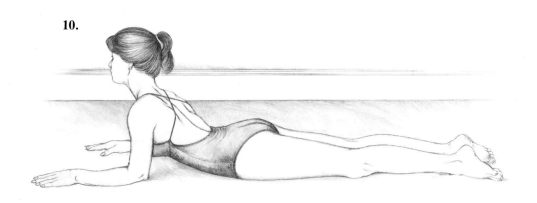

11.

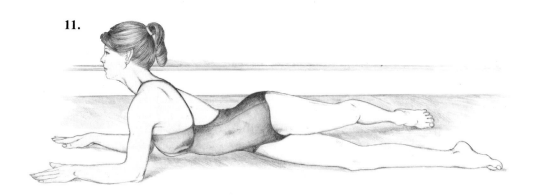

12.   Stand facing the wall with your body almost touching it. Push your pubic bone and thighs into the wall and tighten your buttocks towards each other. Then tightening both sides of your back muscles towards each other drop your head gently back to open your throat, and draw your shoulders together and downwards to open your chest and belly. To avoid discomfort or pain in your lower back make sure that both sides of your back including your shoulders and buttocks are tightening towards each other. Slide your hands down the backs of your legs and make sure that your shoulders and shoulder-blades are moving towards your lower back. Try for five seconds then come up and repeat two or three times.

13.   Kneel on the floor, legs a few inches apart. Come up onto your knees and tighten your buttocks towards each other, your shoulders towards each other and the sides of your back towards each other. Then pushing your pelvis slightly forward take your head back and open your chest and belly by bending your spine. Then grasp your heels. Now make sure your buttocks are tightened together, your pelvis is well forward and you feel no strain in your lower back. If you do not tighten your buttocks sufficiently you will feel strain in your lower back. Hold for ten to fifteen seconds.

14.   Lying on your front place the palms of your hands by your chest at the level of your breast. Tighten your buttocks towards each other, your shoulders towards each other and both sides of your spine towards each other. Take a deep breath in as you take your head and upper trunk forwards and upwards extending and stretching the front of your body and shortening the back of your body. Keep your shoulders and shoulder-blades down towards your lower back as you take your weight on your arms. This is not a press up where your arms do the lifting. Use your spine to extend backwards and your arms as supports. Come down on the exhalation and repeat five times.

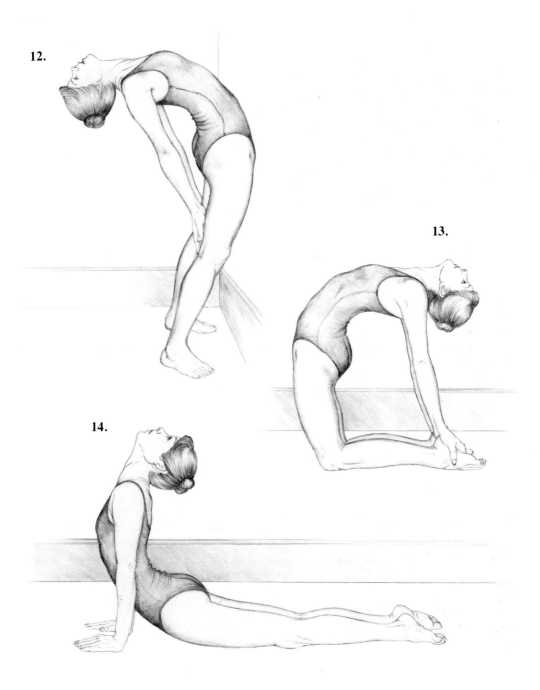

12.

13.

14.

31

15. Lie on your back on the floor. Bend your knees and bring your heels to your buttocks. Grasp your ankles and then tightening your buttocks as hard as you can lift your pelvis as high off the floor as possible. Hold for ten seconds and repeat several times.

16. If your shoulders and spine are supple and you have been practising the other backbending stretches you can then attempt this advanced stretch. This position demands the full lengthening and opening of the front of your body. Lie on your back on the floor, raise your elbows over your head and place your palms under your shoulders, fingers pointing towards your feet. Bend your knees and bring your heels close to your buttocks. Tighten your buttocks towards each other, your shoulders towards each other, and both sides of your spine towards each other. With a deep breath in lift off by straightening your elbows and lifting your pelvis and belly upwards. Rest your head on the floor for a few breaths, then, breathing in deeply again, stretch your arms from your shoulders until your elbows are straight. Relax your head and neck and lift up your abdomen as high as possible by further tightening your buttocks and pulling your shoulder-blades down towards your back. Stay in it for ten seconds. When this is easy push your heels into the floor and slowly push in the direction of your chest and gradually increase the stretch.

15.

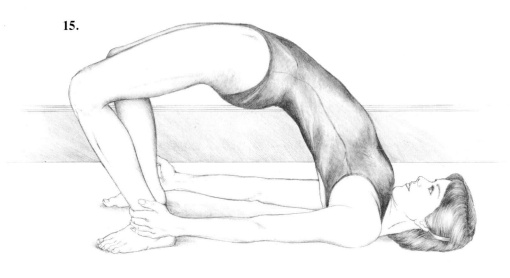

16.

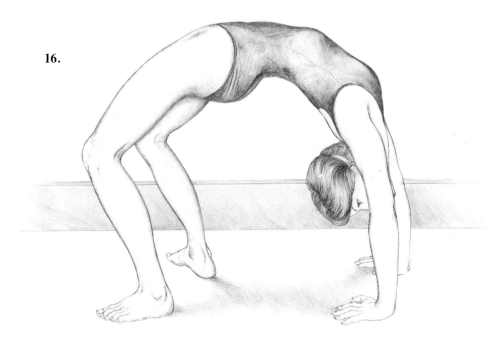

17. Keep your shoulders down as far away from your ears as possible. Drop your chin slightly below the horizontal position. Now take your ear down towards your shoulder making sure the opposite shoulder is anchored well down. As you take your ear down lengthen your neck as much as possible making a wide as possible arc with your head. Feel the stretch on the opposite side. Quick stretch five seconds, long stretch anything up to thirty seconds. Repeat other side.

18. Stand with your feet apart. Let your arms hang with your palms on the sides of your thighs. Let your head drop to the side and then follow with your whole trunk. Make sure your shoulders are down and your buttocks tight. Repeat other side. Quick stretch ten seconds each side, long stretch thirty seconds each side.

19. The same again with the top arm extending over your head and your other arm sliding down your leg. Quick stretch ten seconds each side, long stretch thirty seconds each side.

20. When side stretching is easy try this advanced side stretch. With both arms stretched above your head and with your hands interlocked bend gently but fully to the side making the widest possible arc.

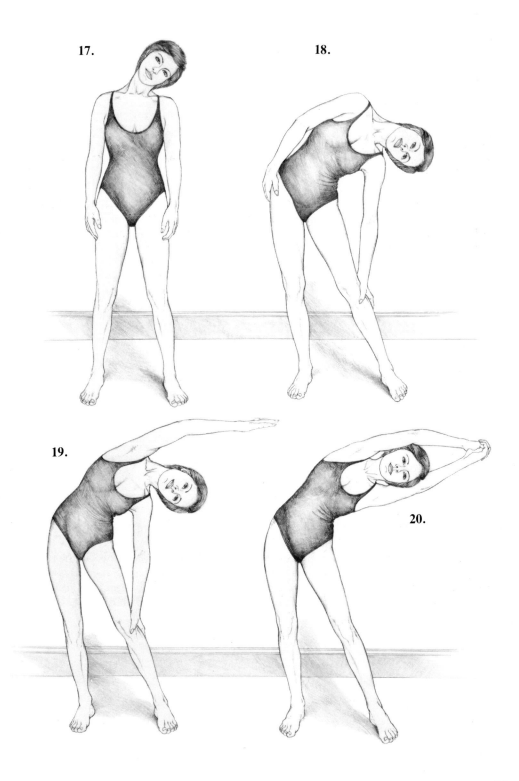

21. Standing or sitting with your arms by your sides, rotate your head to look as far behind you as possible. As you do this consciously draw your shoulders downwards by drawing your elbows downwards. Ten seconds each side and repeat several times.

22. Stand with your back to a wall. Swing round placing your palms on the wall at shoulder width and level with your shoulders. Fixing your arms and shoulders rotate your pelvis, thighs and knees to the front. Make sure your buttocks are tight and your shoulders are down. Hold for fifteen seconds and repeat other side.

23. Lie on your back with your hands interlocked underneath your head. Bend your knees keeping your feet on the floor. Cross one leg over the other and hook the foot of the top leg under the calf of the lower leg. Keep your shoulders down and both elbows on the floor while you take your top knee down to its opposite side by rotating your pelvis. If your elbow lifts up stretch out your arm and hold onto a heavy object like the leg of a table or chair. Hold for thirty seconds breathing smoothly and repeat on the other side. Eventually build up to one minute.

21.

22.

23.

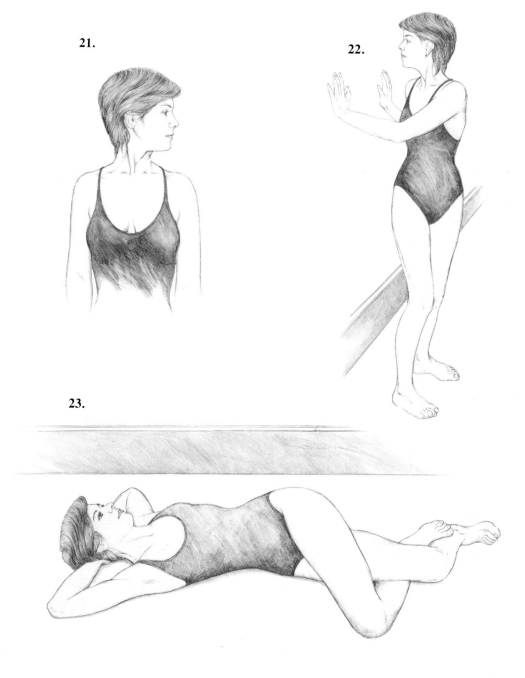

24. Standing or sitting drop your chin onto your chest and interlock your hands on the back of your head just beneath your crown. Allow your arms to hang from your head. Now consciously press your shoulder-blades down towards your lower back. The point is not to pull your arms or raise your shoulders, but to relax your arms and pull down with your shoulder-blades. Again remember to breathe smoothly and you should feel the stretch anywhere between the base of your skull and in between the bottom of your shoulder-blades. Try this stretch for ten seconds and build up to half a minute.

25. Lie on your back on the floor. Arms by your sides, palms down, bend your knees towards your belly. Push on the floor with your palms, swing over onto the back of your neck until your feet touch the floor. If your spine is stiff you may need a cushion or a chair to rest your feet on as they may not touch the floor. Keep your chin well into your chest. You can give yourself extra support by putting your hands on your back and bringing your elbows close together. If this is easy extend your arms and interlock your hands placing your knees on either side of your head. If your knees cannot touch the floor they will eventually with practice. Stay in this position for half a minute and build up to several minutes.

N.B. In these two stretches, particularly the last one, you may find that your breathing feels restricted. Don't worry about it and just relax into the stretch. Your breath will become easy and natural. Any discomfort in your neck or in between your shoulder-blades will ease in time. If you feel discomfort in your lower back take it very easy and slowly and don't push it. This too will go in time. Remember not to force your stretches. Stretch to suit your own body.

24.

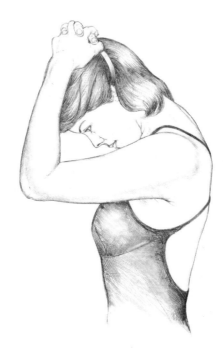

25.

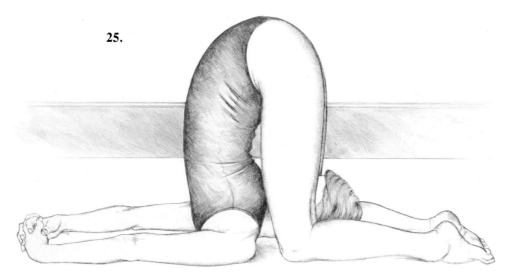

26a.   Stand with your feet a few inches apart. Interlock your hands on your back behind you. Bend forward with your hands joined on your buttocks. Bend from your hips and not from your waist keeping your back straight. Now lift your shoulder-blades lightly towards your hands. This prevents any strain on your sacroiliac and lower back joints. Just hang comfortably and effortlessly. You may also bob gently up and down in this position to increase the stretch. Try half a minute and build up to three minutes.

26b.   To focus the stretch on one leg, simply bend one knee and allow the weight of your head and trunk to stretch out the straight leg. Try half a minute and then repeat other side.

If you are loose in these positions, consciously press your toes into the floor and lift your buttocks as high as you can to increase the stretch even more.

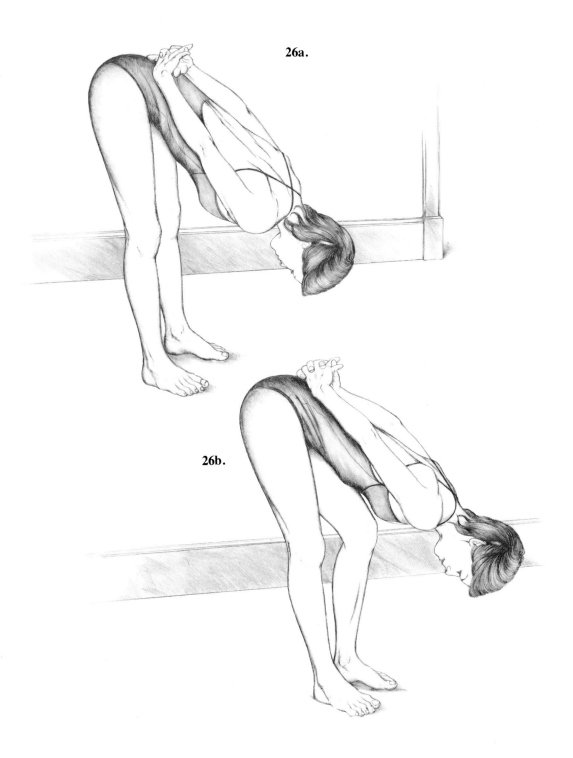

26a.

26b.

41

27. Spread your feet five feet apart, turn your toes in slightly and your heels out slightly. With your hands joined on your buttocks lever your pelvis and trunk forward, bending from your hip joints and not your waist. Just hang comfortably and effortlessly. Keep your pelvis, trunk and head in a straight line. Start with one minute and build up to several minutes.

28. From a standing position, with your feet together, place one foot about three feet in front of the other. Turn your back foot out to about forty-five degrees. With your hands joined behind you on your buttocks slowly bend forward from your hips. Hang comfortably and effortlessly over your front leg. Keep your back straight. Feel the stretch at the back of your front leg. Try half a minute and repeat other side. Eventually build up to two minutes. You may gently bob up and down in these positions to increase the stretch.

27.

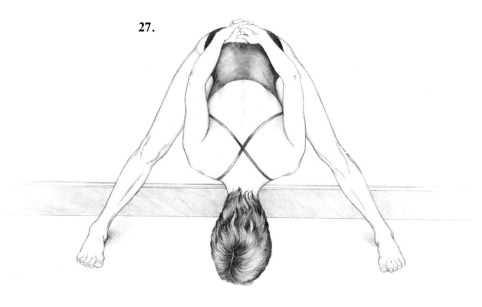

28.

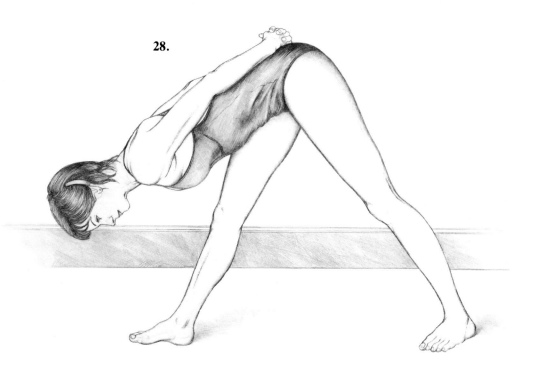

43

29. Stand facing the wall and place your foot on the wall at roughly hip height (this can also be done on a table or low wall). Clasp your hands behind you and keep your shoulders down, standing as erect as possible with both legs straight. This in itself can be a stretch. When this is easy lean your body forward lifting your chest towards your upper leg. Try not to raise your shoulders or bend your back. Feel the stretch at the back of the raised leg. Try half to one minute and repeat on the other side.

30. Starting from the same position bend your raised leg and move your trunk and pelvis towards your thigh. Make sure you keep your lower leg straight. Gently rock your pelvis backwards and forwards and feel the stretch high up in your thigh. Try fifteen seconds and repeat other side.

31. From the same position turn the foot that is on the ground to the side and bend from your hip towards that foot. The raised leg should also remain straight but will also turn to the side as you face to the side. Keep your hands behind you on your buttocks and hang comfortably. Try a half to one minute, then change legs and repeat on the other side.

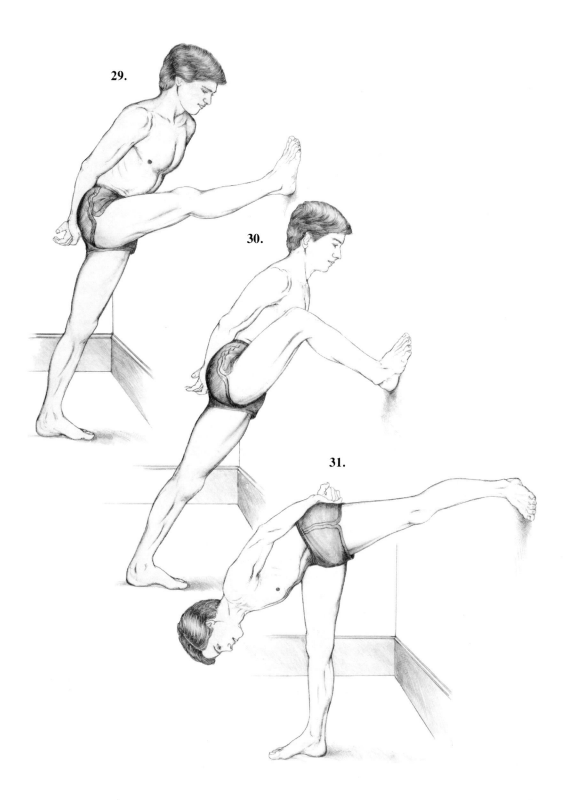

29.

30.

31.

45

32a.   Take a belt or strap and lie on your back with your buttocks and the backs of both legs touching a wall. Loop the belt around one foot and slowly and gently pull the foot down towards your head. Keep your leg straight at the knee. To increase the stretch gradually pull further and further. Try half a minute then change legs and repeat other side. Eventually build up to several minutes on each leg.

32b.   When you feel you are ready try this more advanced stretch. Lie on your back and bend one knee into your chest. Clasp your foot with both hands and straighten your leg. Hold the stretch for half a minute and repeat on your other leg.

33a.   When this last stretch becomes easy try this. Take the raised leg outwards and gradually down to the floor at the side of you. Hold for fifteen seconds and repeat other side.

33b.   From the same starting position with the leg raised, take your foot down to the floor at the other side of you by rotating your pelvis. Make sure both arms and shoulders are touching the floor and both knees are straight. Try fifteen seconds and repeat other side.

N.B.   Stretches 32a, 32b and 33b can all be done in sequence one leg at a time.

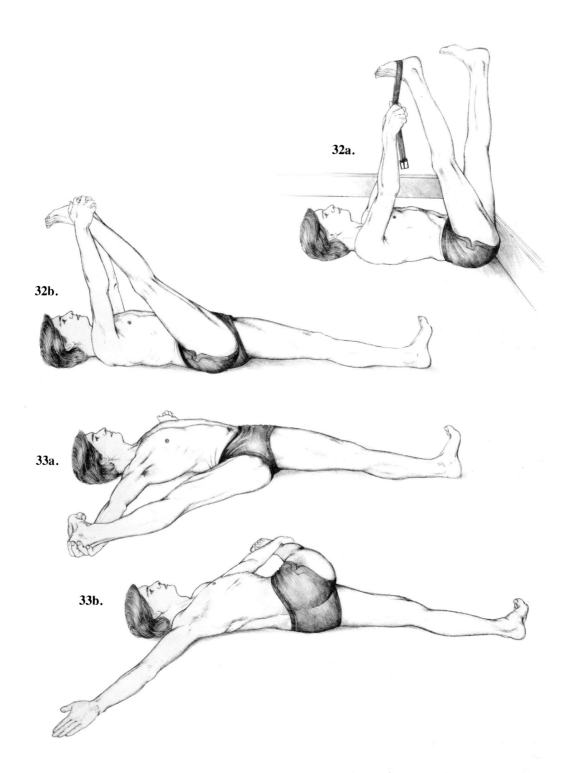

32a.

32b.

33a.

33b.

47

34. Stand facing a wall. Lean onto the wall with your shoulders supporting you at shoulder width and one wrist crossed over the other. Rest your head comfortably where your arms cross. Now bend one knee forward and extend the other knee backwards pushing your back heel down. Keep the toes of both feet pointing forwards, angling your back foot to stretch your calf muscle and Achilles' tendon. Try half a minute and repeat on the other side. You will, after a while, feel a cramp-like pull at the top of your calves. Don't be alarmed at this. Allow it to reach its peak and slowly fade.

35a. Kneeling on all fours place your hands at the bottom of a wall at shoulder width. Come onto your feet and straighten your knees. Pushing your heels to the ground, tighten your shoulder-blades towards each other and expand your chest towards your feet by pushing with your hands. Try half a minute to one minute.

35b. Now bend one knee and take the full stretch on one leg. Try half a minute on each leg.

35c. To increase the stretch from the same position, raise one leg behind you as high as possible pushing the other heel down at the same time. Try fifteen seconds on each leg.

N.B. These stretches lengthen and give elasticity to the backs of your lower legs. The calf muscles are responsible for the spring and bounce in most of our everyday activities. That they are relaxed and supple is most important and cannot be overstressed. These stretches are also noted for the shape and definition they bring to the leg.

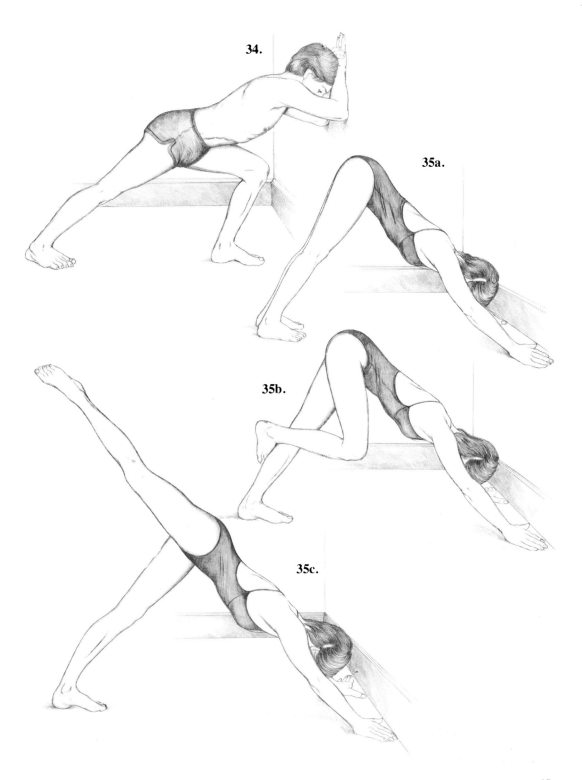

34.

35a.

35b.

35c.

49

36. Stand with your feet about eighteen inches apart, toes turned slightly outwards. Now bend your knees and squat, keeping your knees comfortably apart and your heels flat on the floor. You may need to hold onto something for support. Try one minute and build up to three minutes.

37a. Once you are comfortable in this position without support, stand with your feet only a few inches apart, and squat keeping your knees together, your heels on the floor and your arms extended. Try half a minute and build up to two or three minutes.

37b. If, or when, this is easy straighten one leg out in front of you and clasp your foot with your hands. Balance in this position for fifteen seconds and then repeat on the other side.

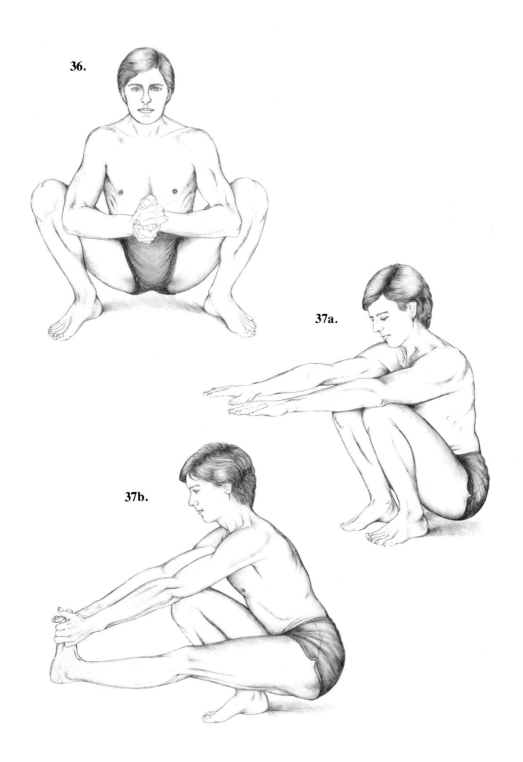

36.

37a.

37b.

51

38.   From the wide squatting position (Stretch 36) lean forward with your weight onto your hands and extend one leg out to the side with the knee straight and toes pointing directly upwards. Now lift your hands off the floor and balance on your bent leg keeping both heels on the floor. Feel the stretch in your groin and thigh. Try thirty seconds and build up to one minute, then go back to the squatting position and repeat on the other side. When this becomes easy you can swing from one side to the other side without moving the position of either heel.

39.   Stand with your hands interlocked behind you and your legs about three to four feet apart and your toes pointing directly forwards. Slowly bend your knees keeping them vertically in line with your feet. Bend at your hips to bring your thighs and trunk horizontal to the floor. In this position extend your chest forward and your shoulders back. Stay in this position from fifteen seconds to half a minute.

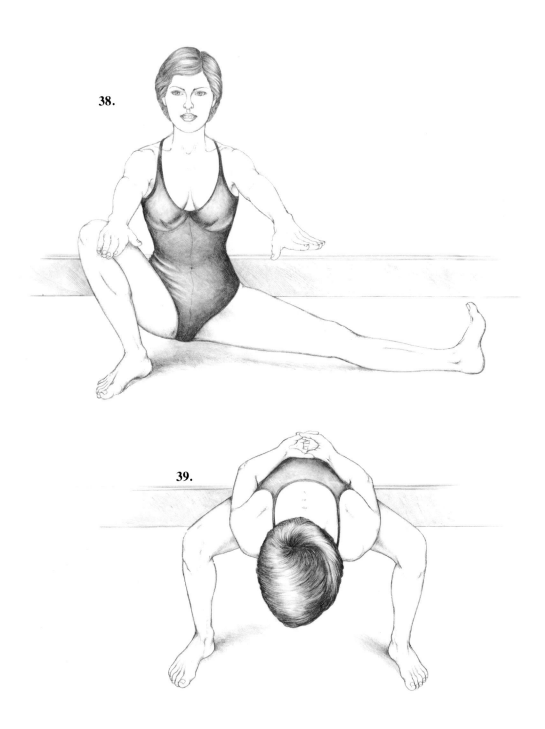

38.

39.

40a.   Sit on your heels with your knees together. Rise up onto your knees and place one leg a few feet in front of you and rest your weight on it. Bring your trunk down onto the inside of your front thigh and place your hand a few inches in front of your foot. Now try to place both elbows on the ground in line with the heel of your front foot. You will feel the stretch in the groin and thigh. Try half a minute and change sides.

40b.   Raise your trunk up again and support your weight on one hand. Bend your back knee and pull your heel in towards your buttock with the other hand. Now push your pelvis towards the ground to stretch the front of your back thigh. At first the sensation in the thigh may feel extreme but with gradual cultivation of this position the initial intensity soon relaxes. Try fifteen seconds to half a minute. Once again remember to breathe smoothly through all the stretches.

41a.   Sit on your heels and come up onto your knees. Stretch one leg out in front of you keeping it straight and support yourself on your hands. Slide your front foot forward as far as you can without too much discomfort. Work into it for fifteen seconds and repeat on the other side.

41b.   Practising this last stretch consistently eventually leads to the full splits. Once this final stretch is cultivated and has become easy you can spend anything up to one minute on each side.

40a.

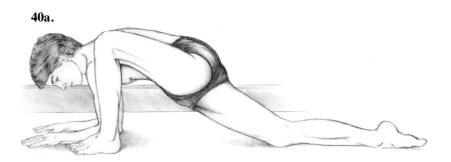

40b.

41a.

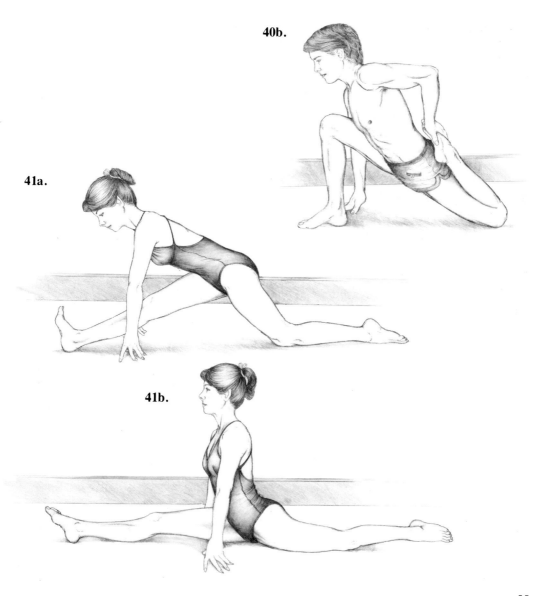

41b.

42a.   Sit with your back against a wall and your legs straight out in front of you. Bend your knees, bring your feet together and pull your heels in as close to your pubic bone as possible. Gently work your knees towards the floor stretching the inside of your upper thighs and groin. If you need to increase the stretch press your thighs down with your elbows or hands, or alternatively slightly raise and drop your knees rhythmically. Spend one minute in this stretch and build up to five minutes.

42b.   Once your knees reach or almost reach the floor, the next step is to clasp your feet with your hands and pull your trunk forward. Try to keep your back straight and lift your buttocks slightly off the floor to come forward. If this is difficult try gently rocking your trunk forwards and backwards from your pelvis. Try working into this for one minute and eventually build up to five minutes. Eventually with consistent practice your belly should come in contact with your feet.

43.   Lie on your back and draw your heels up to your buttocks. Now spread your knees as wide as possible bringing the soles of your feet to touch each other. Tilt your pelvis upwards by tightening your buttocks so that your lower back flattens onto the floor. Stay in this position for one minute and build up to three minutes. For an extra stretch slightly lift and drop your knees rhythmically.

44.   Lie with your buttocks next to the wall, legs up the wall. Straighten your legs and open them gently as far as possible. Keep your knees straight and don't point your toes. Remember not to over stretch to begin with and as always use your breathing to relax into the stretch. Start with one minute and gradually build up to five. Eventually the legs get wider and wider.

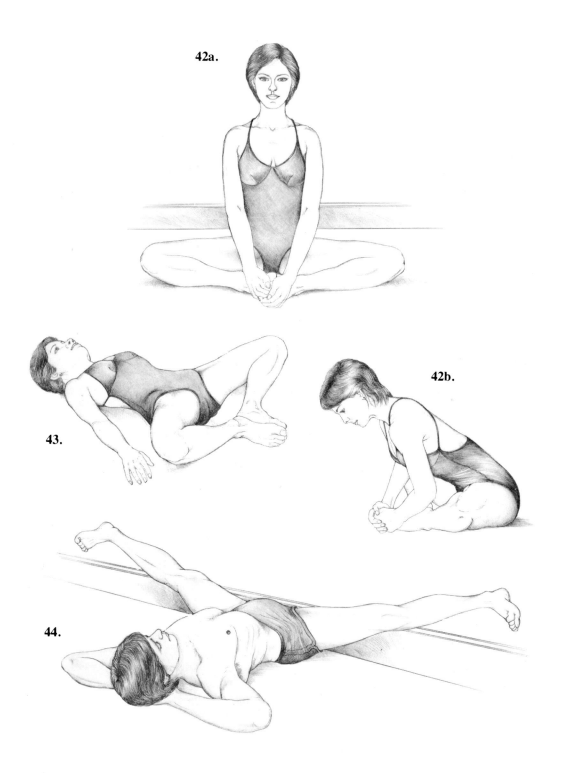

42a.

43.

42b.

44.

45a. Sit on your heels, knees together. Slowly move your feet apart and allow your buttocks to touch the floor. Make sure your toes turn slightly inwards and your heels outwards (See 45b). If this position is uncomfortable place a small cushion under your buttocks. This stretch will make you aware of stiffness in your knees and the front of your ankles. Start with half a minute and build up to several minutes.

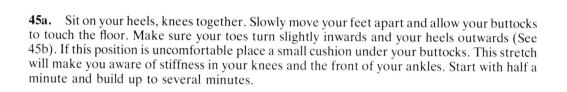

46a. From the same position lean back on your elbows. Tighten your buttocks together and tilt your pelvis upwards to reduce the curve in your lower back to its minimum. Feel the stretch at the front of your thighs. For a quick stretch fifteen seconds, for a long stretch try one to two minutes.

46b. When this last position is easy, keeping your pelvis tilted up and your buttocks tightened, slowly lower your back onto the floor. Stop the movement if you feel any pain in your lower back. If your lower back feels comfortable interlock your hands behind your head. The main stretch should be at the front of your thighs. Try fifteen seconds to start with and build up to a few minutes as it gradually becomes easier.

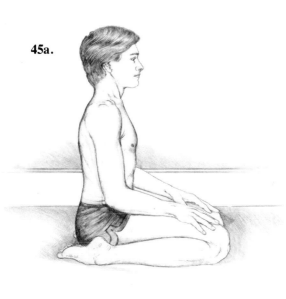

45a.

45b.

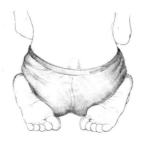

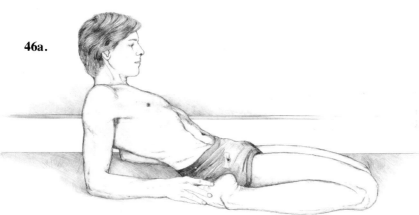

46a.

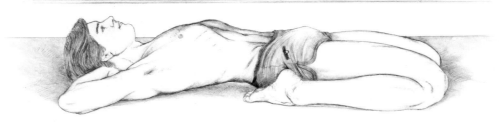

46b.

Your knees are the largest joints in your body. They tend to stiffen up considerably and need stretching regularly and carefully. Many of the other leg stretches will help to loosen up your knees but these stretches are particularly for the knees alone.

47. Sit with your legs stretched out in front of you. Bend one knee and with your hands bring your ankle well up onto your opposite thigh. Slowly and cautiously work your bent knee down to touch the floor, and then in towards your other knee. Try fifteen to thirty seconds on each leg. Don't force your knees, however stiff they seem to be. Time and patience will loosen them.

48. When these preliminary knee stretches are easy, try the full lotus position. Your knees should be as close together as possible and your ankles well up onto your thighs. As this is a difficult stretch, choose your own time and then reverse legs. Never force your knees into this position.

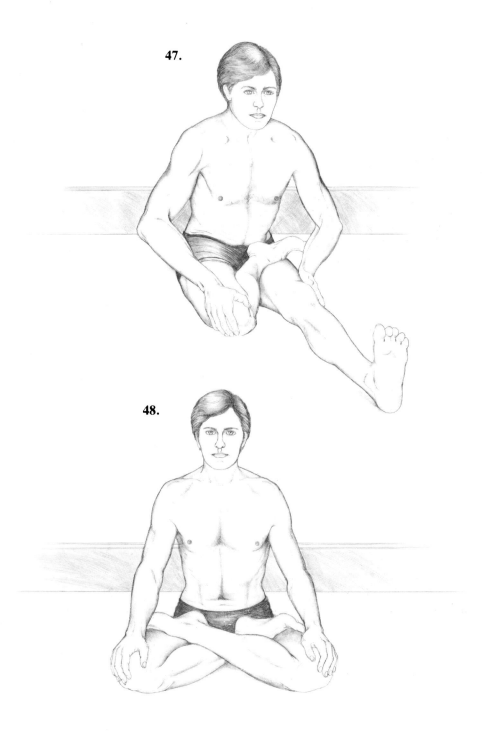

47.

48.

49a. Sit with your buttocks between your feet (See 49b), with your knees open as wide as possible. If you can't sit between your feet, sit on your heels. Quick stretch one minute, long stretch three minutes.

50a. From this sitting position lean forward onto your hands and elbows keeping your buttocks close to your feet. Start with one minute and for a longer stretch build up to three minutes. Try to bend from your hips and not your lower back.

50b. Gradually, in stages, stretch your arms forward until you get the maximum stretch that suits you. If you stretch regularly your chest and belly will eventually reach the floor without your buttocks lifting. Once your chest rests on the floor you can clasp your hands behind your back. Try one minute for a quick stretch and build up to three minutes for a longer stretch. Five minutes is possible with ease once you have cultivated the movement.

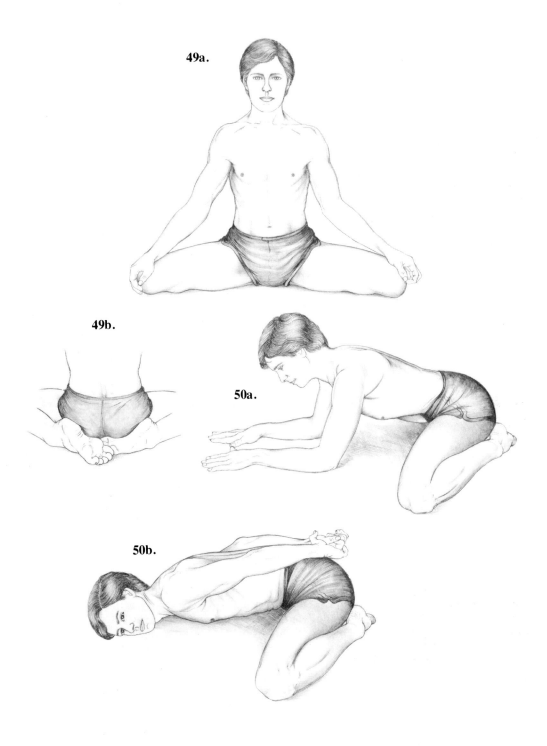

49a.

49b.

50a.

50b.

63

51. Sit on the floor with your legs as wide apart and your back as upright as possible. If you need support to sit upright, put your hands on the floor behind you or sit on the edge of a small cushion. Keep your knees straight and don't point your toes. Remember to use your breathing to ease into the stretch. Try half a minute and for a longer fuller stretch build up to three minutes.

52. When this sitting position is easy rotate your trunk towards either knee and stretch towards your foot. Keep your back as straight as possible, and bend from the hip. If possible clasp your foot to lever yourself down. Hold for ten seconds and then repeat other side. Eventually with much practice your chest and belly will touch down onto your leg.

53. From the starting position (Exercise 51) slowly stretch your hands forward and try to lay your chest and belly on the floor with your back as straight as possible and lifting your buttocks slightly. This final stretch can take a long time to cultivate, you cannot rush it. It is, however, one of the most rewarding stretches once you finally get there. For a quick stretch work into it for thirty seconds and for a long stretch work into it for anything up to three minutes.

51.

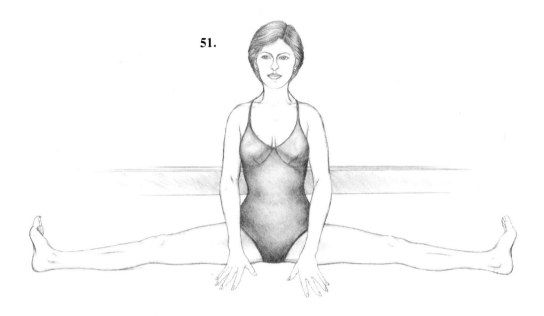

52.

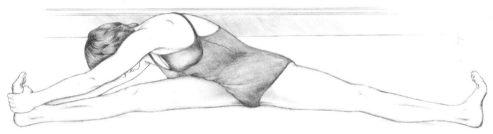

53.

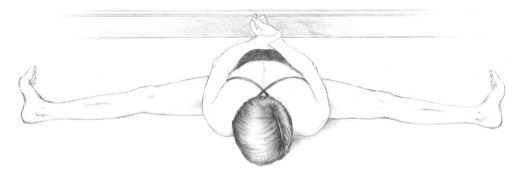

Stretches for the wrists, hands and feet
The extremities of your body, that is your hands and feet, are common sites for stiffness, for arthritic and rheumatic conditions and for trapped or blocked 'body vitality' or energy. If you regularly stretch the joints of your wrists, hands, fingers, feet and toes, you can help prevent painful conditions and increase the vitality level of your entire body.

Wrists
54. Straighten one arm in front of you, palm face up. Rotate your palm outwards from the shoulder, then with your other hand increase the rotation. Hold for twenty to thirty seconds and then repeat on the other arm.

55. Put your palms down on the floor with your fingers facing forwards. Rotate your hands outwards and bring your fingers to face directly inwards towards you. Keep your elbows straight and your palms down on the floor. To increase the stretch move your shoulders backwards, keeping your hands in the same position. This reduces the angle between the back of your hand and your lower arm. Start at thirty seconds and build up to a minute.

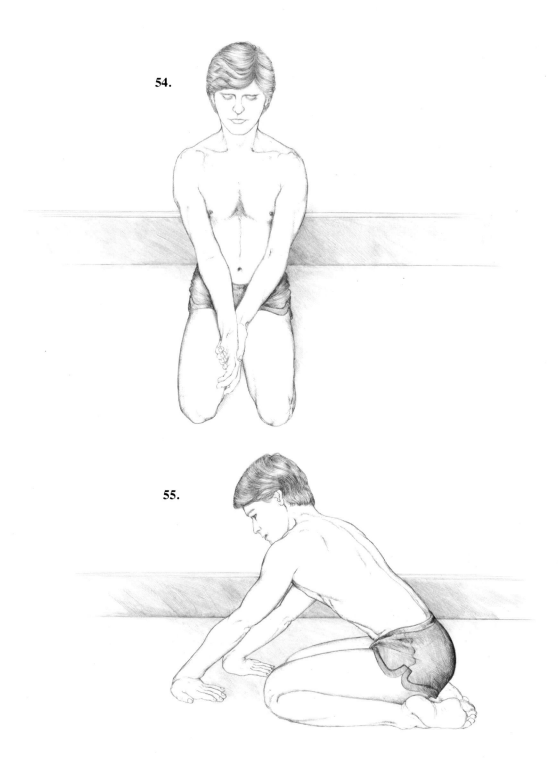

54.

55.

Hands

56a. Rotate each thumb to its limit in both directions.

   b. Rotate each finger to its limit in both directions.

   c. Flex or bend each of your knuckle joints in turn.

   d. Bend each of your middle finger joints forward to their limits.

   e. Bend each of your top finger joints to their limits.

   f. Bend your wrist and thumb downwards towards your lower arm.

   g. Extend or bend backwards each of your top finger joints.

   h. Extend or bend backwards each of your fingers in turn, extending all three of your finger joints to their limits.

Hold all these stretches for five to ten seconds each.

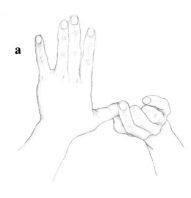 a

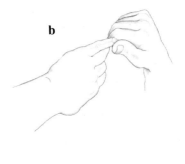 b

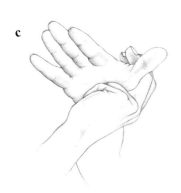 c

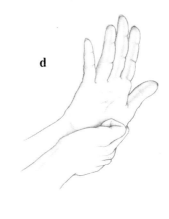 d

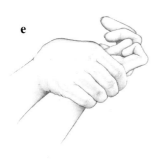 e

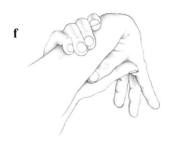 f

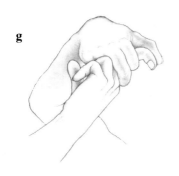 g

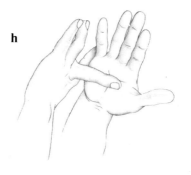 h

Feet
57a.   Spread your toes apart by separating first your big toe from your little toe, and then each toe in turn.

   b.   Pull each toe in turn, creating space between the joints.

   c.   Stretch each toe backwards. This will also stretch the underneath of your foot.

   d.   Bend the top and the middle joints of each toe forward.

   e.   Rotate each toe in both directions.

   f.   Using your fingers and the palm of your hand, bend all the toes except the big one forward.

Hold all these stretches for five to ten seconds each.

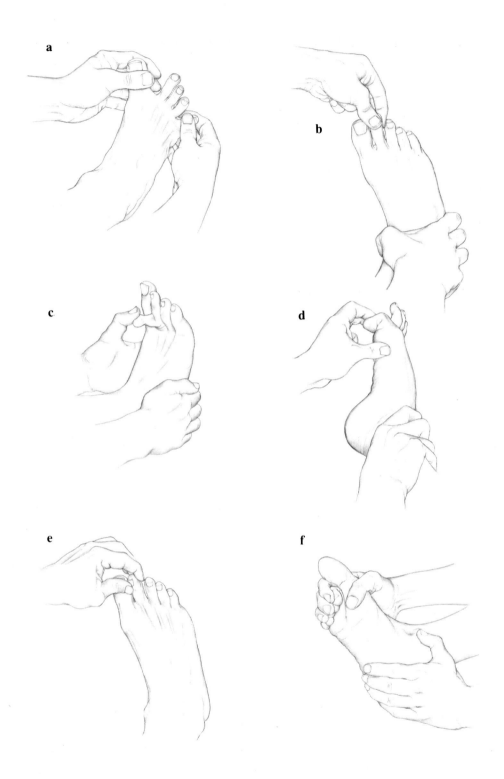

71

7. Manipulation and Partner Stretches 1 – 27

Manipulations, whether osteopathic, chiropractic, medical or bone-setting, are used as a kind of first aid, that often gives relief from pain in a relatively short period of time. A manipulation is mostly used when a person's joints and muscles are in some state of distress or injury.

Of all the people seeking manipulative therapy roughly 52 per cent do so because of lower back pain, 20 per cent because of neck pain, 13 per cent because of other spinal problems and 7 per cent because of headaches. Most of the remaining 8 per cent have problems with the joints of their limbs. Pain is the main reason for wanting treatment.

Manipulations are a form of stretching, as manipulative techniques fundamentally stretch the soft parts of the body by pushing joints to their extreme limits. They increase mobility. However, the direct aim of manipulation is not necessarily to restore full range to a joint at which limitation exists. It is mostly directed to making the existing limited movement painless instead of painful – that is to say, to restore pain-free stiffness. Whereas the aim of soft stretching exercises is eventually to restore full range to joints, to dissolve stiffness as much as possible.

Back and neck pain is also approached differently. The human trunk is like a strung bow, the spinal column is the bow and the abdomen, breast and front are the string. Manipulations focus most attention on the bow. They concentrate on adjusting individual vertebrae to relieve pain. These quick adjustments often relieve pain but they do not radically increase mobility to the extent that it alters the patient's posture.

Soft exercise or stretching on the other hand focuses attention on the string. The reasoning behind this is that to whatever extent the string (belly, chest, and abdomen) is loosened and relaxed, the load on the bow (spinal column) will be lessened. Regular stretching, unlike manipulations, noticeably and radically increases mobility and alters posture. It relieves back pain, neck pain, and other musculo-skeletal pain, not by focusing on individual spinal vertebrae, but by focusing on every joint of the body and particularly by stretching, relaxing and opening up the belly, throat and shoulders.

Soft stretching exercises are ideal to use and cultivate after the first aid of professional manipulation.

All the stretches of chapter 6, i.e. performed regularly, are excellent remedial exercises after manipulative techniques have released acute or chronic pain and injury. However, to increase the effect of these stretches after you have become reasonably familiar with them, you can be helped by working with a partner. The following stretches for two are a kind of non-professional series of manipulations. Non-professional means that no study and expertise is needed by you or your partner.

Partner Stretches

Partner stretches should begin when both partners are to some extent familiar with the individual stretches. Partner stretches increase the power of stretching and should be practised only when both partners want to exceed the limits they can reach individually. Each partner stretch has instruction for the person being stretched and for the person assisting. Both partners should follow the instruction carefully as these stretches are most effective when performed correctly. Here is a general guide for both partners.

72

When being stretched get into the appropriate position, relax and breathe normally for several seconds before your partner begins to assist you. If you cannot remember how to adopt a stretching position, simply refer back to the same exercise shown in chapter 6. In most of the stretches your partner uses leaning weight to stretch you. If you sense any unnecessary muscular effort or force coming from your partner, you should say so. When being stretched consciously try to let go of resistance in the area being worked by breathing smoothly and evenly. If you need more or less of a stretch indicate this so that your partner may adjust his or her weight appropriately. If you wish a stretch to be held at a particular point then say so. The amount of time given to any particular partner stretch is up to you. If your partner is highly sensitive to your muscular responses and uses a very slow and gradual approach, some of the stretches may be held for a minute or more. However, for most people ten to thirty seconds is usually ample for an effective stretch.

When assisting a partner make sure that your partner is in the correct position and comfortably relaxed before you begin to assist. It is important that you yourself are relaxed. With most of these stretches you are merely using your body weight and you need very little muscular force or effort. As with the individual stretches, your main tool is gravity. Follow the instruction carefully as to how and where to apply your weight or assistance. By having practised the individual stretches you will have some idea of the location and nature of the sensations felt by your partner. Always apply your weight slowly and gradually without putting your partner through any unnecessary stress. *Give the stretch to suit your partner by checking his or her responses at all times.* Breathing should be smooth and even. If you are in a position to observe your partner's face, note its expression, it should remain calm and relaxed. Fulfil any wish your partner may express for more or less of a stretch, or for a stretch to be held at any particular point. You will learn to sense your partner's muscular responses. You may feel them either tensing up under your hands or melting passively further into the stretch. Ease up if your partner tenses up against you. If more of a stretch is required apply more weight on your partner's exhalation, this way your partner is not working against you. At first someone may tense up against a stretch but may be unaware of it themselves. Stretching individually and with a partner teaches you about physical resistance. It not only teaches you how to let go of your own resistances but also how to help another let go of theirs. The amount of time stretching a partner is arbitrary. It depends on various factors like how stiff or supple your partner may be, the nature of the stretch, how much time you have, and so on. The more sensitive you become to your partner's responses the longer you will be able to assist them in any particular stretch if desirable. There are no suggested timings, hold the stretch to suit your partner. As soon as your partner indicates that they have had enough then stop the stretch immediately.

PARTNER STRETCH 1

When being stretched

a.   Keep your elbows straight and your hands at shoulder width.
b.   Lift your chest towards the wall and keep your shoulders and shoulder-blades drawn down towards your lower back.
c.   Make sure your partner's assistance is not forced but relaxed and that you feel weight leaning on you and not a pushing pressure.
d.   Make sure your partner's line of force is downwards along your back and not upwards and forwards.
e.   Make sure your partner does not lean too heavily onto your lower back. Most of the emphasis should be along your spine as far down as the lower ribs.

When assisting

a.   Transfer your weight from directly above that part of your partner's spine you are leaning on. The direction of your weight should be downwards and away from your partner's head – a pull downwards.
b.   Keep your contact arm straight at the elbow and apply your weight gradually.
c.   Make sure the soft fleshy heel of your hand is used for contact with your partner's spine.
d.   Tune into your partner's breathing or any sign of undue stress and allow him or her to guide you verbally.

PARTNER STRETCH 2

When being stretched

a.   Do not lift your shoulders towards your ears, keep them down.
b.   Make sure your arms are shoulder width apart.
c.   Your assistant should take you gradually to your limits by edging your hands away from your body.
d.   Make sure you are in control of how far you want to go.

When assisting

a.   Gently and gradually extend your partner's arms and stop immediately you are told to.
b.   Grip your partner's wrists firmly but gently.
c.   Maintain your partner's arms at shoulder width throughout the stretch.

1.

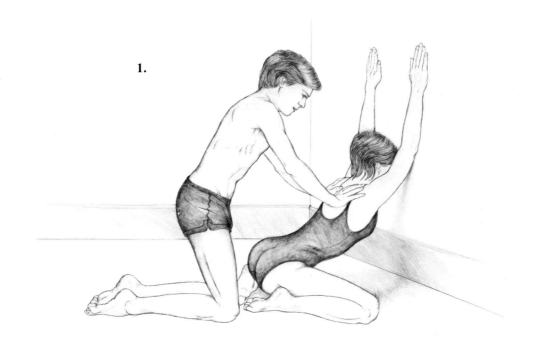

2.

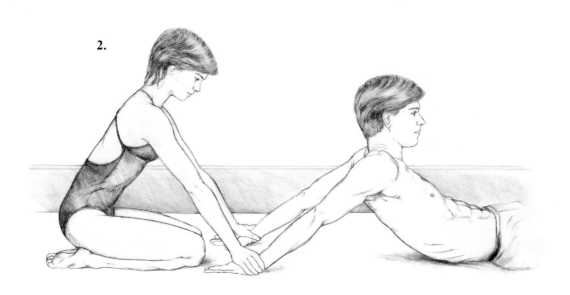

75

PARTNER STRETCH 3

When being stretched

a.   Place your hands on the sides of your waist with your thumbs and fingers pointing forwards.
b.   Keep your shoulders drawn down towards your feet.
c.   Don't push your head forward.
d.   Keep a straight spine but relax and breathe normally.

When assisting

a.   Bring your partner's elbows gently but firmly towards each other.
b.   Be aware of your partner's resistance and note the breathing. If you feel a strong resistance to your movement and any increase in your partner's breathing rate, ease off and start slowly again.

PARTNER STRETCH 4

When being stretched

a.   Keep your shoulders drawn downwards.
b.   Your fingers, palms and arms should be extended to their limits making as large an arc as possible.
c.   Don't push your head forward.
d.   Remember to give your partner feedback as to how you would like the stretch, and to use your breathing to help you let go of any specific sensations of tightness.

When assisting

a.   Make sure your partner's shoulders do not rise, and that his or her palms and fingers are extended fully.
b.   Grip your partner's elbows and gently pull his or her arms backwards and at a slightly upward angle.
c.   Go so far back until your partner signals you to stop.

N.B.   One may feel these stretches at the back or front of the shoulders and chest or both.

3.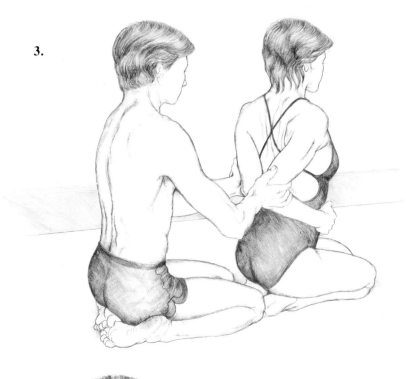

4.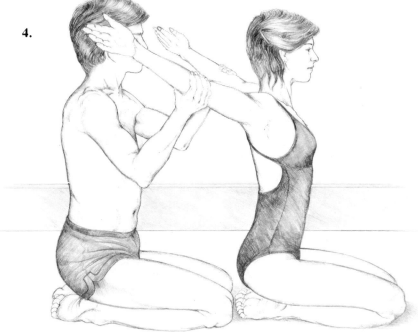

PARTNER STRETCH 5

When being stretched

a. Keep your back erect.
b. Make sure your hands are firmly linked.
c. Breathe smoothly.
d. Don't arch your back.

When assisting

a. Position the elbow of your top arm onto the back of your partner's shoulder. Using your elbow as a lever, pull your partner's raised elbow backwards, downwards and slightly inwards.
b. Use your other hand to pull your partner's lower elbow backwards, inwards, and upwards.

N.B. You are in effect drawing your partner's elbows together through a diagonal line across their back.

PARTNER STRETCH 6

When being stretched

a. Make sure your head and back are erect.
b. Try to get your fingers as high up your back as possible with your palms together.
c. Keep your shoulders drawn downwards.
d. Breathe and relax as your partner draws your elbows backwards and more closely together.

When assisting

a. Don't force your partner's elbows back with too much muscular effort. Gradually and gently pull the elbows backwards and closer together.
b. Remember to use your partner's exhalation to increase the stretch.
c. Note your partner's responses, sense the resistance and stop when signalled.

N.B. Remember there are no suggested timings. The person being stretched should decide how long the stretch should last.

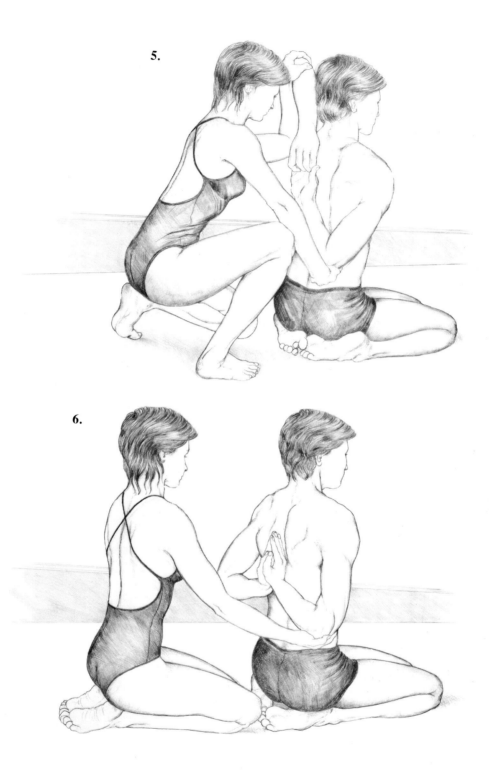

5.

6.

PARTNER STRETCH 7

When being stretched

a.   Place your elbows well forward and a few inches apart.
b.   Cup your hands well under your chin.
c.   Keep your shoulders down away from your ears.
d.   Slightly tighten your buttocks together.
e.   Gently drop your head back.
f.   Feel the stretch mainly in the throat and upper chest.

When assisting

a.   Place the fleshy heel of one hand on the upper part of your partner's spine with the other palm on top of that.
b.   Gently lean your weight directly downwards.
c.   Work all along your partner's spine.
d.   Apply your weight to synchronise with your partner's exhalation. Check your partner's responses and stop when signalled.

N.B.   The most important point is how you direct your weight. It must always be downwards to shorten your partner's back.

PARTNER STRETCH 8

When being stretched

a.   Place your elbows shoulder width apart with your upper arms vertical to the floor.
b.   Lift up and lengthen your chest and the front of your body while drawing your shoulder-blades back and downwards.
c.   Slightly tighten your buttocks together.

When assisting

a.   Work your partner's middle and lower back.
b.   Have the heels of your hands touching each side of your partner's spine with your fingers pointing directly outwards.
c.   Lean your weight gently and increase it on your partner's exhalation.
d.   Apply your weight through two straight arms. The line of force should be downwards.

N.B.   If the person being stretched feels discomfort in the lower back it means your buttocks are not drawn tightly enough or your partner is leaning too heavily. Both of these exercises are designed to iron out any kinks in the spine and open up the front of the body.

80

7.

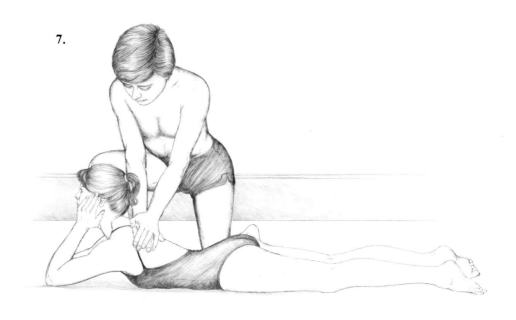

8.

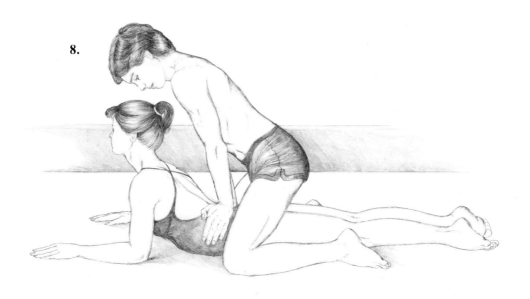

PARTNER STRETCH 9

The full back-bend as mentioned in chapter 6 is one of the most important movements the body is capable of making. There is no other movement that stretches the front of the spine and front of the body to such a degree. This is an advanced stretch and can take a long time to cultivate fully. Assistance in this particular stretch is invaluable in reaching the final goal.

When being stretched   Stage 1

a.   Lie on your back with your head resting on the floor in between your partner's feet.
b.   Bend your knees to bring your heels close to your buttocks but keep the soles of your feet flat on the floor.
c.   Extend your arms over your head and firmly grasp your partner's ankles with both hands.
d.   Tighten your buttocks slightly and pushing your feet firmly into the floor lift your pelvis as high as you can, with your head resting on the floor.
e.   Breathe easily in preparation for the next stage. So far you have extended your lower trunk hips and thighs. If you feel any discomfort in your lower back at this stage you are not ready for the next stage.

Stage 2

f.   Keeping your buttocks tightened as firmly as possible, straighten your elbows to lift your head off the floor and to raise your chest as high as possible. At this point your partner will begin to support you at your shoulders.
g.   Make sure your hands grip your partner's ankles firmly, that your elbows are fully straightened and that your head is hanging freely. Keep your shoulders and shoulder-blades drawn away from your head to shorten your back as much as possible. Again make sure that your buttocks are firmly tightened to support and protect your lower back.
h.   If this is easy press down on your heels, lifting your toes off the floor. At the same time open your chest, throat and belly to their maximum by tightening your buttocks more firmly together, tightening your back muscles together and rocking your chest towards your partner's legs.
i.   This partner stretch emphasises the stretching of the shoulders and eventually the upper chest.

When assisting   Stage 1

a.   Stand with your buttocks against the wall, your feet at shoulder width and about 9 inches from the wall.
b.   Make sure your partner grasps your ankles firmly and is positioned centrally with their head between your feet.
c.   As your partner starts to lift off, bend your knees by sliding your buttocks down the wall and lean your trunk forward until you can give full support with your hands on each of your partner's shoulder-blades.

Stage 2

d.   As you take your partner up into the stretch let your legs do most of the work by straightening them out slowly and leaning your trunk back towards the wall. In other words make sure you are positioned economically in terms of your own effort.
e.   Do not pull your partner into a full stretch but give enough support to allow him or her to make the movement without strain. Check your partner's responses and lower slowly to the floor when he or she has had enough.

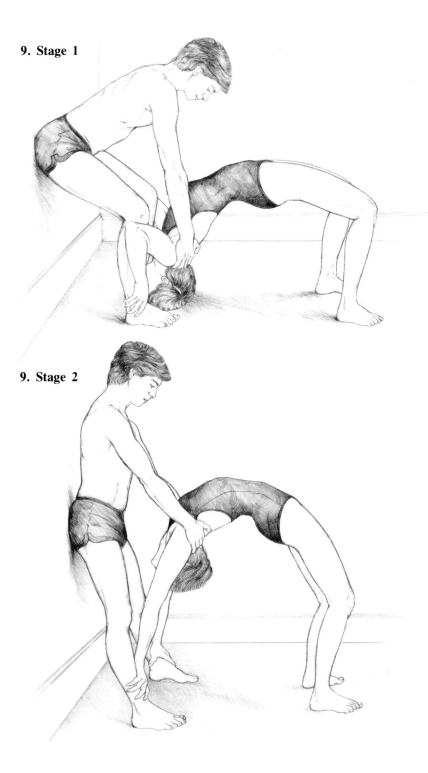

9. Stage 1

9. Stage 2

83

PARTNER STRETCH 10

When being stretched

a.   Stand with your back to the wall with your heels about 9 inches from it. With your hips facing forward twist your upper body round and place your palms shoulder height and shoulder width apart, firmly on the wall.
b.   Do not lift your shoulders, keep them drawn downwards.
c.   When your partner turns your hips forwards, resist the movement from the waist up by keeping your upper body steadily fixed to the wall.
d.   Repeat other side.

When assisting

a.   Place your hands on both your partner's hips.
b.   Gently and steadily turn your partner's pelvis to the front sensing your partner's resistance.
c.   The leverage on both hips should be as equal and even as possible.
d.   Repeat other side.

PARTNER STRETCH 11

When being stretched

a.   Lie down in the appropriate position and make sure you are completely passive and relaxed.
b.   When your partner rotates your hips keep breathing smoothly and evenly.
c.   Remember to guide your partner by saying what you are feeling, whether you want more or less weight, or whether you want the stretch held at a particular point.
d.   Repeat other side.

When assisting

a.   Use your foot to anchor your partner's elbow firmly and gently to the floor.
b.   Place one hand on your partner's knee and the other at the back of your partner's hip.
c.   Lean your weight slowly onto your partner's knee and at the same time with an equal and even force rotate your partner's hips. Remember to keep the elbow anchored to the floor.
d.   Your partner will most probably feel the stretch in the front of the shoulders, or around the belly and chest, or in the lower back. Wherever the stretch is experienced pay attention to your partner's face and breathing in order to gauge his or her limits.
e.   Repeat other side.

N.B.   When being stretched, if you cannot remember how to adopt a particular position then refer back to the instruction for that position in chapter 6.

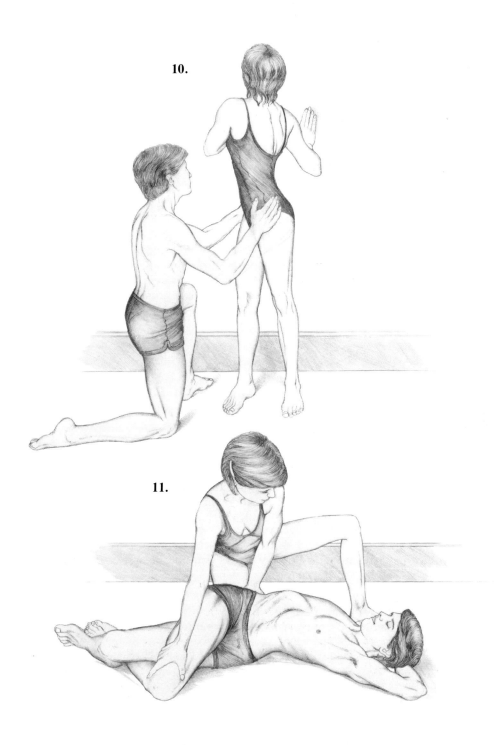

10.

11.

85

PARTNER STRETCH 12

When being stretched

a. Lie face up on the floor, bend your knees and relax.
b. When your partner lifts your head make sure it feels well supported and your chin is in a central position.

When assisting

a. Slightly depress the tips of your partner's shoulders with the soles of your feet.
b. Ease up close so that you can easily and comfortably cradle the back of your partner's head in the palms of your hands.
c. Taking the head firmly but gently, slightly lengthen your partner's neck and take the head upwards and forwards.
d. Once you have your partner's head well up and forwards, you can position your elbows against the inside of your knees to help you support the weight and apply more leverage. The more relaxed and comfortable you are yourself the easier it will be to sense the tension and resistance in your partner's spine, neck and shoulders.
e. Hold your partner in this position, sense the resistance, tune into the breathing, and increase or stop the movement at your partner's wish.
f. Lower your partner's head slowly to the floor.

PARTNER STRETCH 13

When being stretched

a. Simply roll over onto the back of your neck with your knees by your ears and your arms extended out behind you.
b. Interlock your fingers and take a few breaths to relax into the position.
c. Consciously and with the help of your breathing allow your partner to rock your pelvis gently to and fro while holding your hands firmly on the floor. Feel the stretch in the upper back, neck and shoulders.

N.B. This stretch in particular must be easy before you use the assistance of a partner.

When assisting

a. Anchor your partner's hands to the floor.
b. With your other hand on the back of their pelvis gently rock your partner to and fro to increase and reduce the stretch alternately.
c. A very slight push forward is all that is needed. It is a matter of pushing and catching, pushing and catching.
d. As usual pay attention to your partner's breathing, resistance and any wish they may express to alter or stop the stretch.

12.

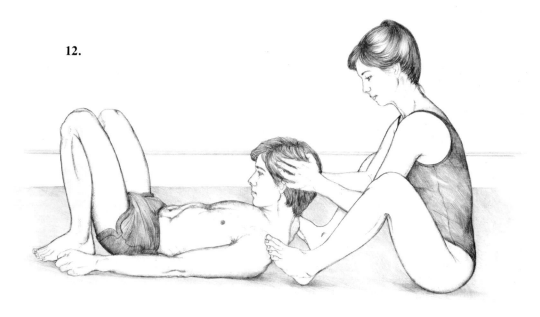

13.

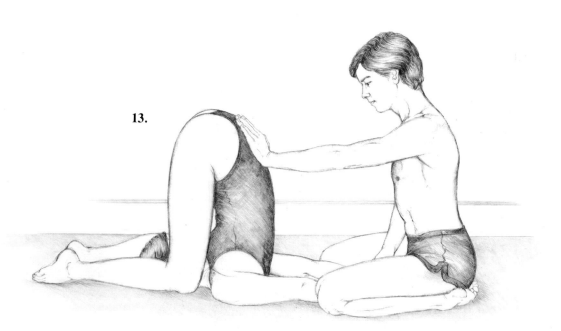

PARTNER STRETCH 14

When being stretched

a.   Lie on your front and relax completely. Keep your shoulder-blades drawn gently down.

When assisting

a.   Anchor your partner's pelvis to the floor by gently leaning your weight on the upper part of their buttocks.
b.   Lift your partner's leg and bend the heel in as closely to your partner's buttock as is comfortably possible.
c.   Repeat other side.

N.B.   This is an elementary stretch for the front of the thigh and knee. Some may be able to make the movement easily and not feel much of a stretch. On the other hand it may take some time before the heel comfortably touches the buttock

PARTNER STRETCH 15

When being stretched

a.   Lie back in this position and tighten your buttocks.
b.   Uptilt your pelvis to reduce the curve of your lower back to its minimum.

When assisting

a.   Place one hand on the front bony part of your partner's pelvis just by the hip. Place your other hand on their knee. Slowly lean your weight to anchor the pelvis down and gently take the knee to the floor.

N.B.   Because the muscles at the front of the thigh are attached to the pelvis and the pelvis is attached to the lower back these stretches are fundamental in reducing an accentuated lower back curve. This is an example of how muscles seemingly unrelated to the spine can affect its integrity.

14.

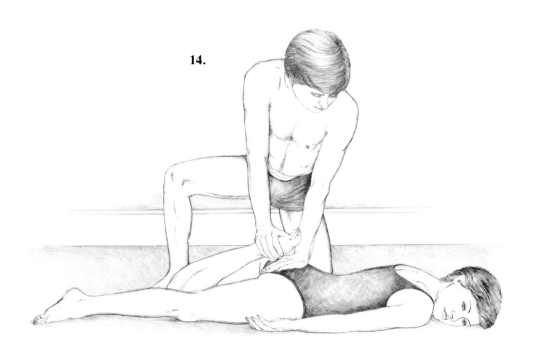

15.

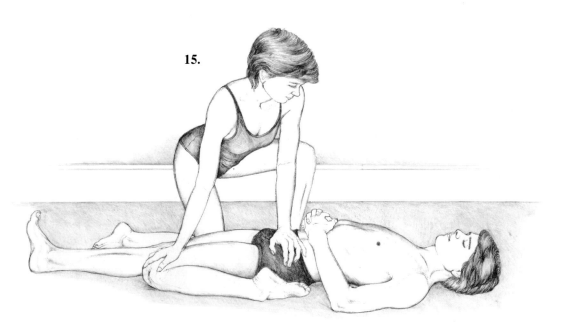

89

PARTNER STRETCH 16

When being stretched

a. Lie down face up and feel as comfortable and relaxed as possible.
b. Bend one knee in towards your chest.
c. Breathe smoothly and evenly as your partner takes you into the stretch.

When assisting

a. Anchor the leg down firmly on the floor with one hand just above the knee.
b. Gradually apply your weight through your hand resting on your partner's bent knee.
c. Stop your partner's thigh from falling sideways by supporting it with your front leg.
d. Equalise your weight through both of your arms keeping them straight at the elbow.
e. Check your partner's responses.
f. Repeat other side.

N.B.   This stretch is useful in detecting any imbalance between the hip joints. Most people have one hip that is to some degree stiffer than the other. Stretching regularly in time evens out the differences.

PARTNER STRETCH 17

When being stretched

a. Lie down face up and relax.
b. Bend one knee to your chest and straighten the leg.
c. Keep your raised leg straight at the knee and the toes pointing down towards you.
d. Breathe smoothly and consciously try to let go of any sensations of tightness in your hamstrings and calf muscles as your partner stretches you out.

N.B.   Remember when being stretched it is you that should be in full control of how far you want to go.

When assisting

a. Anchor your partner's thigh down to the floor just above the knee by using your own knee.
b. Anchor the thigh down just firmly enough to keep it on the floor, don't be too heavy.
c. With one hand lean onto your partner's heel to take it closer to their head.
d. With your other hand just above your partner's knee pull back to keep the leg as straight as possible.
e. Distribute the opposing forces of both your arms equally.
f. As usual check your partner's responses and repeat other side.

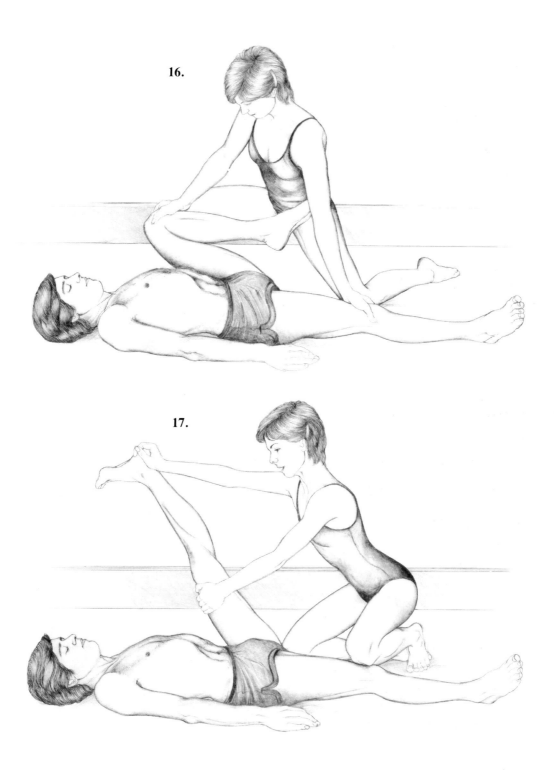

16.

17.

PARTNER STRETCH 18

When being stretched

a.　Keep the back of your pelvis right into the wall and your body as upright as possible.
b.　Keep your heels pulled closely to your pubic bone.
c.　As you feel your partner's weight on your thighs, consciously allow your knees to sink slowly down towards the floor.
d.　Feel the stretch on your inner thighs and groin and direct your partner as to how you would like the stretch.

When assisting

a.　Place your hands well onto your partner's thighs a few inches in from the knees.
b.　As you lean your weight, distribute it evenly through both your arms.
c.　If one thigh opens more than the other, adjust your weight appropriately.
d.　Check your partner's responses, sense any resistance.

PARTNER STRETCH 19

When being stretched

a.　Keep your buttocks close to the wall and your body as upright as possible, but leave enough space for your partner behind you.
b.　Consciously relax your thighs completely to the floor.

When assisting

a.　Stand behind your partner and support yourself on the wall before you position your feet.
b.　Gently place your feet on your partner's thighs a few inches in from the knees.
c.　Make yourself as light as possible by leaning back against the wall and slightly bending your knees.
d.　Stop immediately your partner indicates he or she has had enough.

N.B.　This last stretch is obviously for people who are already quite open in this movement. It should be tried when the previous stretch has become relatively easy.

18.

19.

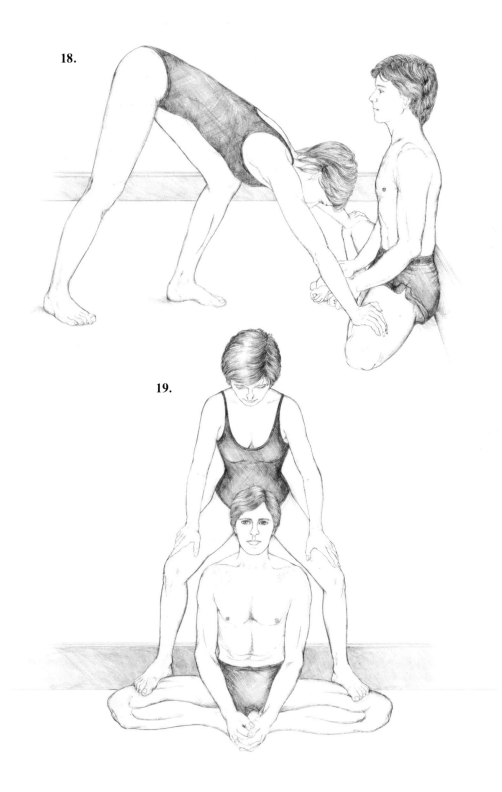

PARTNER STRETCH 20

When being stretched

a.   Lie on your back and draw your feet as close to your pubic bone as possible.
b.   Bring the soles of your feet to touch each other by turning your feet in and your knees outwards.
c.   Allow your knees to drop to the side keeping your lower back on the floor. You can use a cushion under your feet to ensure your back stays on the floor.
d.   As your partner applies weight to your knees tighten your buttocks and tilt your pubic bone upwards to reduce any exaggerated curve in your lower back.
e.   Remember to breathe smoothly.
f.   Eventually both knees reach the floor.

When assisting

a.   Apply weight very gradually and evenly onto your partner's knees.
b.   Direct your weight forwards and downwards. Directing it downwards and backwards causes your partner to arch the lower back.
c.   Remember to keep your arms straight.
d.   Tune into your partner's breathing and resistance, and stop when signalled.

PARTNER STRETCH 21

When being stretched

a.   Lie on your back with your hands underneath your head.
b.   Bring one ankle to rest on the other leg just above the knee, and relax.
c.   Make sure you feel comfortable and guide your partner as to how you would like the stretch.

When assisting

a.   Anchor your partner's pelvis down on the side of the straight leg.
b.   Slowly apply your weight onto your partner's bent knee with your other hand.
c.   Gradually take the knee down towards the floor and as you apply the weight through both your hands get the feeling of spreading them away from each other.
d.   Check your partner's responses, stop when signalled and repeat other side.

N.B.   Two kinds of sensations may be felt in these stretches. Most common is the feeling of stretch at the front of the hip and inner thigh. Less common is the sensation of the soft tissue shortening and closing at the back of the hip. You may feel one or both of these sensations. Whichever use your own feelings to guide you and tell your partner when to ease off when necessary or stop completely.

20.

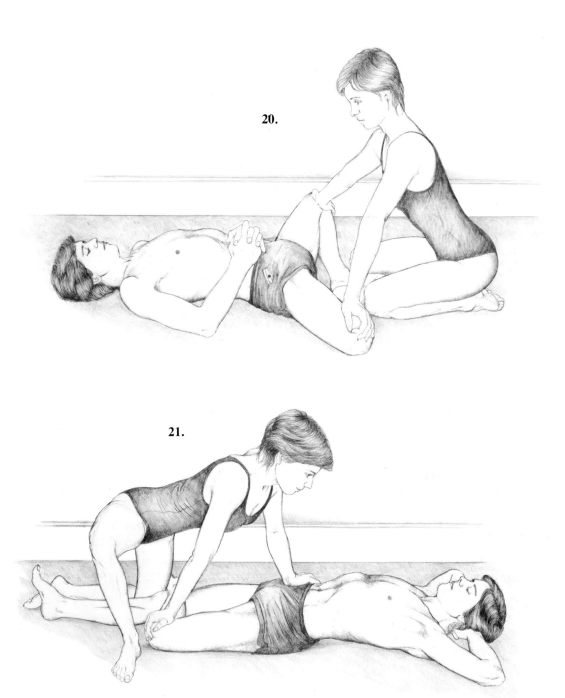

21.

PARTNER STRETCH 22

When being stretched

a.　Keep your buttocks as close to the wall as possible.
b.　As your partner leans on your thighs go with the weight by allowing your knees to sink closer to the floor.
c.　Remember to guide your partner to exactly the force you need.

When assisting

a.　Place your hands on your partner's knees, relax your body, and keeping your arms straight lean forward effortlessly.
b.　If one leg feels stiffer than the other adjust your weight accordingly.
c.　Increase the weight on your partner's exhalation.
d.　Check your partner's responses and stop when told.

PARTNER STRETCH 23

When being stretched

a.　Stretch your knees as wide as possible.
b.　Don't worry if your buttocks lift off the floor.
c.　Keep your shoulders drawn backwards away from your ears to shorten your upper back slightly.

When assisting

a.　Make sure that your hand leaning on your partner's sacrum is transferring most of your weight.
b.　The direction of the weight at this point should be down and back towards your partner's feet.
c.　The direction of weight at your front hand should be in the same direction, i.e. a pull towards your partner's feet.
d.　Keep your partner's pelvis anchored well down with your back hand and keeping both arms straight gradually and evenly distribute your weight, i.e. backwards and downwards towards your partner's feet.
e.　If you need to apply more weight, do so on your partner's exhalation.

N.B.　This last position sometimes shows up excessive curvatures or slight humps along your partner's spine. Find the highest point along the spine and use the weight of your front hand to straighten it out slowly. If your back is rounded and protruding it is not the fault of the back but is due to tightness in the groin causing the spine to compensate.

22.

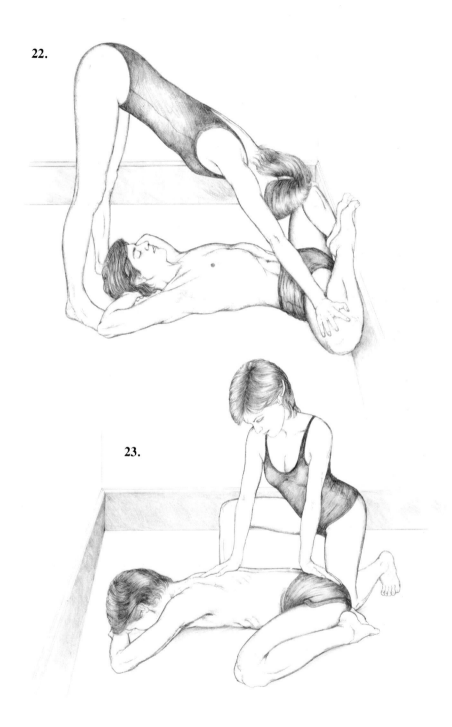

23.

97

PARTNER STRETCH 24

When being stretched

a.   Lie back in this position, tighten your buttocks firmly together and tilt your pubic bone upwards.
b.   Make sure your partner's weight feels evenly distributed through both your hips.
c.   Enjoy the stretch in the front of your thighs and knees, breathe smoothly and indicate when you have had enough.

When assisting

a.   Apply your weight evenly through both your partner's hip bones, keeping your arms straight as you lean.
b.   Use your legs to hold your partner's knees closely together.
c.   The point of applying weight to the pelvis is to reduce the lower back curve to its minimum. The lower back never completely touches the floor, but is at its safest when the curve is at its minimum.

PARTNER STRETCH 25

When being stretched

a.   From the same position keep your buttocks slightly tightened, draw out one leg and allow your bent knee to be levered towards you.
b.   You will feel the stretch in your leg that is positioned on the floor.

N.B.   This is one of the best stretches for the quadriceps and in time reduces exaggerated lower back curve and pain.

When assisting

a.   With one hand anchoring your partner's knee to the floor gently lever the raised leg towards the chest.
b.   Use your front leg to prevent your partner's leg from falling outwards.
c.   Do this very gradually as the sensation in the thigh can be sharp.

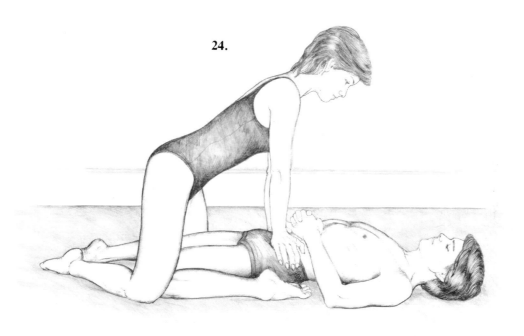

24.

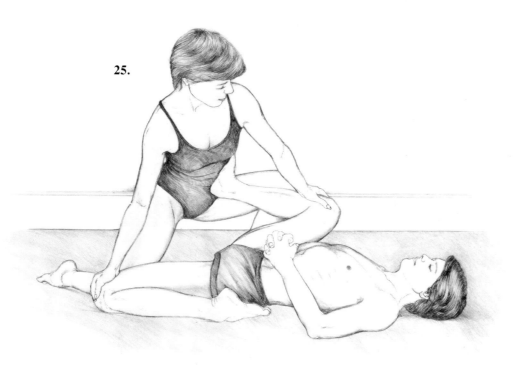

25.

PARTNER STRETCH 26

When being stretched

a.   Squat with your heels on the floor and your body leaning straight back on the wall.
b.   Relax and allow your knees to be taken forwards and away from you.
c.   When your knees are taken forward, don't lift your heels.

When assisting

a.   Simply lean your weight onto your partner's knees to take them forwards and downwards away from your partner's chest and towards their toes.

N.B.   This stretch is especially suitable for those who cannot squat comfortably on their heels.

PARTNER STRETCH 27

When being stretched

a.   Keep your knees as straight as possible.
b.   Keep your elbows straight and at shoulder width.
c.   Shorten your back by drawing your shoulders up and backwards towards your buttocks.
d.   Feel the stretch in your calves and indicate when you have had enough.

When assisting

a.   Place your thigh centrally along your partner's back.
b.   Gently lean your thigh along your partner's back. Use the length of your thigh to lean and not the point of your knee.
c.   Check your partner's responses at all times.
d.   This stretch lengthens the calf muscles and the sensations can be quite acute, so be gentle and gradual.

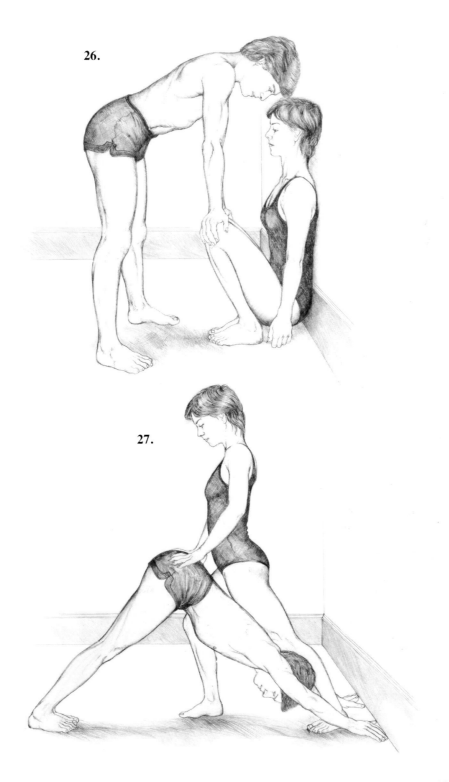

26.

27.

101

8. Stretching Relieves Pain

As the cultivation of stretching directly improves the functioning of your body's musculo-skeletal system, it also prevents headaches, backaches, and most forms of arthritis and rheumatism. Stretching's preventative capacity is obvious. However, its usefulness as a pain reliever seems less obvious.

Gentle stretching over time relieves painful muscles, tendons and joints, generally and specifically.

Arthritis and Rheumatism

Most forms of arthritis and rheumatism are related to stiffness in some way. Stiffness in your joints and muscles is either a symptom or an early warning sign of arthritis or rheumatism. If you suffer from this kind of disorder and the condition is not inflammatory, you can get relief by very carefully and very gently cultivating the stretches of chapter 6. As painful joints and muscles are usually very limited in their range of movement you should merely hint at the stretch and gradually increase the range of movement step by step. There are cases of elderly people who have managed with perseverance to break through their arthritic stiffness and by keeping up their stretching routine achieved a great deal of relief. It is advisable to seek the consent of your doctor, osteopath, chiropractor, acupuncturist or whoever has been treating you before you start stretching.

Headaches

It is common knowledge to medics, osteopaths and chiropractors that more than 80 per cent of all headaches are accompanied by tense, stiff (unrelaxable) head, neck and shoulder muscles (Diagram 7).

The following stretches aim specifically at relaxing the tense muscles that contribute to headaches.

Backache

The root cause of most backaches is not in the back itself. Although it is the back that is strained and feels in pain and discomfort the root cause of most backache arises from the front of the body, namely, from soft parts like the throat, breast and belly as well as thighs and buttocks. Your throat and belly are the most vulnerable parts of your body, they are highly sensitive and have the greatest amount of pain receptors. Because of this there is a natural tendency of the body to overprotect these areas. The body normally does so by assuming subtle protective postures that close up the front of the trunk and put strain on the back. Most backache is the result of poorly balanced muscle pulls on the trunk, head, shoulders, pelvis and thighs.

The following stretches concentrate on correcting these muscle pulls giving more elasticity to the front of the body, thereby alleviating strain and tension in the back.

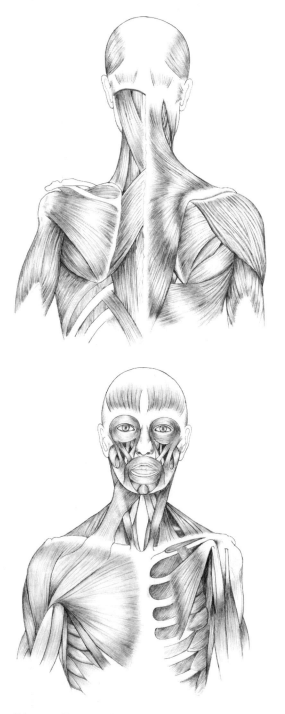

Diagram 7.   Muscles associated with headaches.

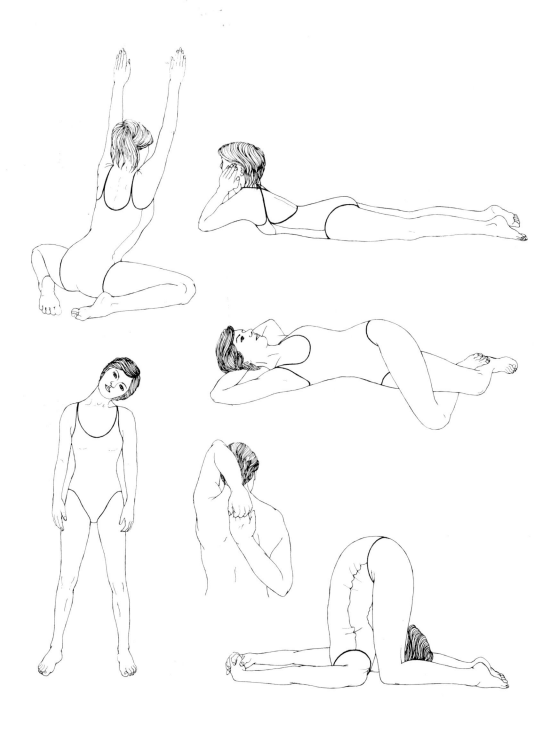

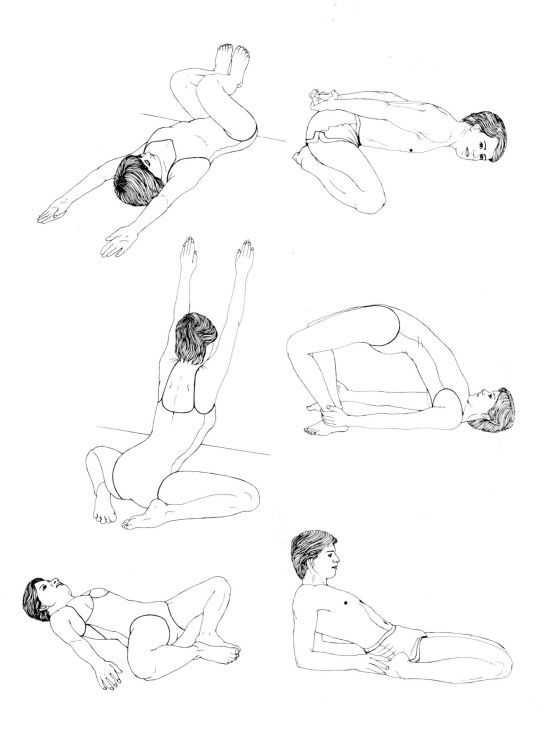

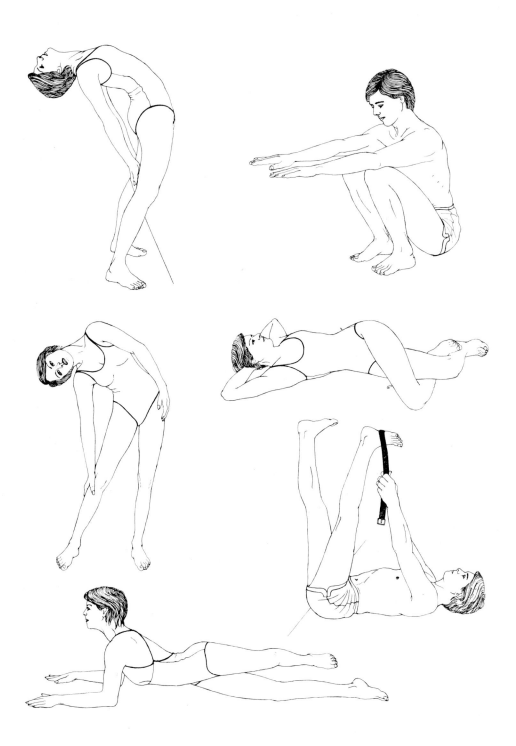

9. Stretching for Sports

Besides sports like gymnastics, diving and figure skating most other sports do not demand a high degree of suppleness and so can and are played with the body quite stiff. However, that is not to say that suppleness is not desirable. The question is how much better could you play your sport, whatever it is, with your body more supple than it is at present? Sebastian Coe, holder of two world records, when asked if he thought he could run still faster answered in effect that that would depend, working with his trainer, on how free and light his spine could be made. And to make the spine freer and lighter, it has to be made more flexible and supple. Stiffness as stated on page 3 is a kind of physical heaviness and a subtle drain of one's energy.

The constant use of stiff joints over the years hastens their wear and tear. For example in competitive sport you have a great tennis player like Lew Hoad and one of the world's best golfers, Lee Trevino. Both were plagued with stiff, painful backs and both eventually had their vertebrae fused to relieve the pain. This is not to say that hard sport is not good for you. Running or playing squash with a reasonably supple body is nourishment for its muscles and joints, its heart and lungs. With very stiff ankles, knees and hips it hastens their deterioration and lays the foundation for such disorders as arthritis and rheumatism. Stretching all your body parts as suggested in chapter 6 improves the flexibility of your major joints and the suppleness and elasticity of the major muscles and tendons of your body. The suppler you are all-round the better you will play your sport without unduly hastening the wear and tear of your body.

Stretching complements hard exercise and sport for many reasons. We have already said that by improving the elasticity of your muscles you automatically improve your breathing and your circulation. You become more physically relaxed, lighter, and more energetic. Benefits like these are obviously an asset to any activity. However, most important is the condition of your muscles and joints themselves.

Stiffness, for someone who regularly jogs, plays sport or practises hard exercise, has other disadvantages. Stiff joints and tight muscles and tendons are more vulnerable to injury than if they were flexible. Stretching regularly, therefore, gets your body in a condition of suppleness that makes it less prone to injury and strain.

Whatever sport you play specific joints and muscles are active more extensively than others. Muscles and other connective tissues are far less likely to strain if they have been stretched and physically relaxed beforehand. To avoid injuring these joints and muscles they can be loosened and relaxed through stretching before and after playing. The following stretches are before and after routines for specific sports.

The stretches given for the following sports/activities complement the movements most common to those sports/activities, and are best suited to the environment peculiar to each activity. We have suggested partner stretch routines for the team sports. However, in order to achieve overall, all-round flexibility, remember to use and cultivate all the stretches of chapters 6 and 7.

Stretching and Running

Running is an activity and sport in itself, and is also common to many other activities and sports. It is a main feature in any activity involving an athletic performance in locomotion, and, as mentioned earlier, running is the perfect example of hard exercise as opposed to the soft, passive exercise of stretching. The two complement and enhance each other. For these reasons it is particularly necessary to explore the benefits that stretching gives to the runner.

Added flexibility and elasticity increase muscle resilience, economise on precious energy, add ease and speed in running, and prevent injury. *Muscle resilience* is dependent upon the elastic quality of muscle tissue. Unlike synthetic elastic which can only stretch and return to its normal position and shape, muscle-tendon tissue can both stretch and shorten and return to normal. It has a two-way resilience. For example, when the ankles are fully flexed and then fully extended, all the muscles and tendons of the ankles have stretched and shortened to their maximum. When you stretch a group of muscles statically you are also shortening its opposing group statically. You are maintaining and building up muscle resilience. Resilience is elasticity, the power for muscle-tendon tissue to resume its original shape and position after shortening, stretching (compression), or lengthening (expansion). Muscle resilience has a dramatic influence on a runner's overall health and fitness. *Stretching influences the energy of a runner*, first by improving elastic energy, secondly by changing the relationship of the body to gravity, and thirdly by improving ease and speed in running.

Elastic Energy
The precise timing of hip, knee, ankle and arm movements allows a runner to make use of the elasticity/resilience inherent in muscle tissue. Because stretched and shortened muscles rebound to their original length, they have the capacity to do free work (no use of energy) and so increase the power and efficiency of movements. Some physiologists believe that elastic/resilient energy may produce as much as half the total energy needed to run. Failure to make muscles supple and resilient, to make the most of this free, inherent elastic energy, is highly wasteful.

Running and Gravity
The body of the runner, like any other body, is a structure that is subject to the force of gravity. When any structure is out of line with this force, gravity puts added strain upon it. You can prove this for yourself by standing upright, feet together, and slowly inclining your body forwards. You can feel the muscles at the back of your legs stiffen to stop you falling forwards. Your body uses up more energy to hold it upright and move it when it is out of line with gravity. A stiff body is a body carrying an unstable load, is out of line with gravity, and is loaded with extra strain. The goal of stretching regularly is to balance the opposing muscle pulls at every joint so that one's body gradually and involuntarily lines up with the force of gravity. Stretching the muscles in this way balances the body at all its joints, automatically improves body stability, therefore conserving valuable energy needed for performances in running.

Stiff joints demand more force, they increase the force that the propulsive muscles need to move the limbs through their range of movement. A well-hinged door needs less force to open and close it than a stiff one. Distance running is a repetitive activity involving countless movements of the joints, and even a slight tightness will restrict leg movements and require extra force to move them through the desired range. Seemingly slight inflexibilities may become substantial over the duration of a run and drain valuable energy. Stiff ankles, knees or hips demand more force and therefore more energy to move them continually and repeatedly at the required rate. Removing stiffness by stretching regularly enables the runner to liberate the inherent energy that is locked up in keeping muscles stiff.

Ironing out Structural Faults
There is no doubt that continued impact against the track or ground when running can lead to a reduction in the range of movement and can compound any existing faults/imbalances in those joints mostly used. When the muscle-tendon units of the runner are fully resilient they can effectively recover and balance out between successive impacts. Because stretching improves the relationship between the opposing teams of muscles that govern every joint it

108

improves the structure, posture and movements of the body as a whole. It alters the arrangement of the parts of the body and lessens the mechanical strain on the weight-bearing joints. For example, the relationship between the hip, knee and ankle joints can be improved by using the appropriate stretching exercises. Many runners who are clearly inadequate vehicles subject themselves to super timing, i.e. high quality repetitions in the hope that they will achieve better results. Stretching daily builds a better machine and so ensures that these repetition sessions bring worthwhile results. An all-round stretching programme practised daily is instrumental in eliminating and reducing many of an athlete's structural deficiencies.

What Muscles need to be Stretched for Running?

A runner needs to increase strength and resilience in the locomotive muscle groups of the legs, thighs, and hips, particularly the quadriceps of the front of the thigh and the gluteals or buttock muscles. This contributes to better leg speed. And as muscles work in opposing teams the antagonists of these main propulsive muscles – the hamstrings need to be made as resilient as possible.

In running, *when the advancing leg is lifted* the lower quad, the upper hamstring and the gluteals are lengthened and stretched and the upper quad and lower hamstring are shortened and contracted; *when the back leg is extended* the reverse happens – the lower quad, the upper hamstring and the gluteals are shortened and contracted and the upper quad and lower hamstring are lengthened and stretched.

To understand which muscles are used and how they are used in running, two simple facts have to be taken into account. First of all, muscles work in opposing groups and secondly that the large muscles of each thigh work two joints, the knee and hips, so that in flexing the knee and hips together and in extending the knee and hip together one part of the quads shortens and the other part lengthens. And so too with the hamstrings. This means that in running these muscles never have both parts fully shortening or lengthening.

Athletes need particular flexibility in

> ankles – flexion and extension
> knees – flexion and extension
> hips – flexion and extension

These six joints need to be able to flex fully and extend fully, to avoid injury and save energy and to increase speed.

The propulsive muscles – those of the lower limbs – need to be made strong and resilient. The shoulders need to be as free floating as possible and the remaining postural muscles need to be well balanced in their pulls on the spinal column, chest and head, to tolerate the stress brought about by the propulsive muscles, shoulder movements and breathing. An economic postural stability is needed. The better balanced the posture of the head, neck, chest and lower trunk, the less energy is needed to keep them stable.

The propulsive muscles of the hips and legs, the shoulder-girdle muscles, and the postural muscles, form three distinctive parts in a runner's stretching routine.

Stretching and Arm and Shoulder Action

Arms and legs work in synchronisation in running. The rhythm of the arms and the rhythm of the legs are obviously interacting. The arms and shoulders play a major role. They don't just hang there. Leg speed, stride length and tempo are all dependent on the upper body. Runners need a degree of fluency and flow so that arm action is rhythmical. Without the action of the arms the trunk would have to twist back and forth to balance the movement of the legs. Efficient arm action keeps the trunk square.

As the arms swing the shoulder-blades should not rise up towards the neck. They should rotate on a fixed axis and not move up and down. Supple shoulders allow the arms to be carried low and relaxed. Stiff, tense shoulders encourage the arms to be carried too high making fluid arm swing (or action) impossible and often resulting in rigid arm carriage which is responsible for shoulder sway and waste of energy.

Runners frequently complain of a tightening and cramping of the deltoids and trapezia muscles, which act as stabilisers of the shoulder-joint and shoulder-girdle while running. This tightness wastes energy and encourages surrounding muscles to contract. The trapezia are large muscles running across the upper back and attached to the collar-bones and back of the head. The trapezia often tighten when the runner maintains a head and neck position in which a curve or hollow spot is formed in the back of the neck. Runners who have postural deviations such as round shoulders and a forward head often develop trapezia tightness.

Tightness can be decreased by gently letting the chin drop towards the chest and then straightening the neck.

Rounded-shouldered runners should stretch their chest and shoulder muscles by grasping a doorway and leaning forward through the door. Exercises which strengthen these muscles should be avoided. Rather the rhomboid muscles located between the shoulder-blades should be strengthened. With greater strength they will tend to pull the shoulder-blades together and keep them firmly against the rib-cage. The result is a stretching in the front of the chest and shoulders and a reduction in the roundness of the shoulders and the forward curved neck.

A full stretching routine practised every day can improve and remove postural deficiencies like round-shoulders, hollow-neck and sunken-in-chest. Supple, well-balanced shoulders and arms are a great asset to any runner.

Sebastian Coe and His Stretching Routine

George Gandy is a lecturer in physical education at Loughborough University and is the trainer of Sebastian Coe, world record holder and Olympic gold medallist. He writes: *'Stretching exercises are, in my view, an absolute must. All the athletes I work with are encouraged to stretch habitually as part and parcel of their daily life. I believe the benefit to be gained relates closely to the amount of time spent in extreme stretch but not stress positions.'*

Unfortunately life's natural processes seem to set strength against mobility losses. Crash programmes for strength may therefore accentuate a decrease in the range of movements of which you are capable. This can be so detrimental to a runner as to negate completely progress in other aspects of fitness. Lack of mobility may also predispose an athlete to injury.

Sebastian Coe's programme of stretching exercises has included work on all main joints. The emphasis, however, has been on ankle flexion and extension, hamstring extensibility, hips' extension and low back mobility in the locations most relevant for a runner.

All routines involve static positions with a feeling of slight stretch — discomfort beyond a minimal level is considered counter-productive. Generally, each position is held for 30 seconds at a time or, with progressive decreases in joint angle, for three consecutive periods of 6–10 seconds. The exercises are advised for at least one hour every day.

Once or twice a week, some 20 minutes or so of partner-assisted stretching is carried out at Loughborough. This is mainly aimed at improving the flexibility of the hamstrings on the back of the thighs.

Best Warm-up and Warm-down

Running experts constantly suggest to beginners that they don't skip a proper warm-up and warm-down. They advise warming up before a run by doing gentle stretching exercises and starting the run slowly. And at the end of the run to do a liberal amount of stretching once again. A regular and proper warm-up sequence can reduce the resistance of muscles and connective tissues to joint movements, assist flexibility, prevent injury and add speed. While an adequate warm-down sequence prevents going to bed feeling stiff or waking up stiff the next day. A stretching programme should begin and follow each run emphasising flexibility of the muscle groups which tend to be tightened by running: calves, hamstrings, quads, lower back and hip flexors. Ten to fifteen minutes of stretching after a run can make a significant difference in how a runner feels the next day.

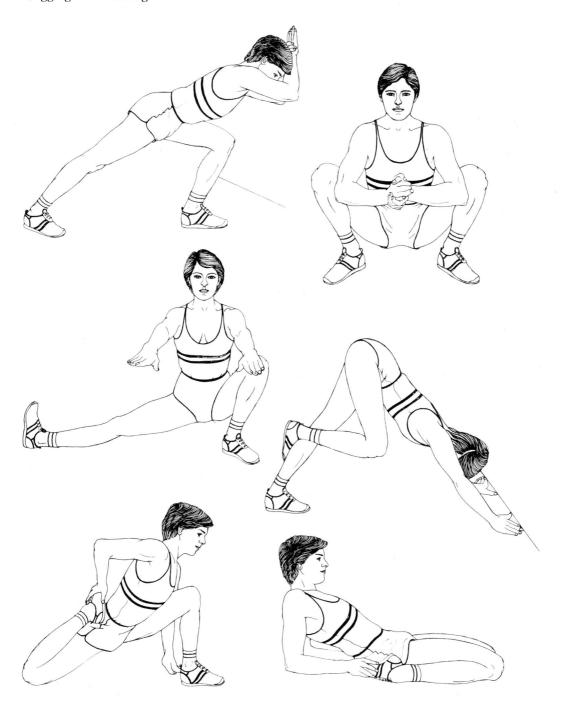

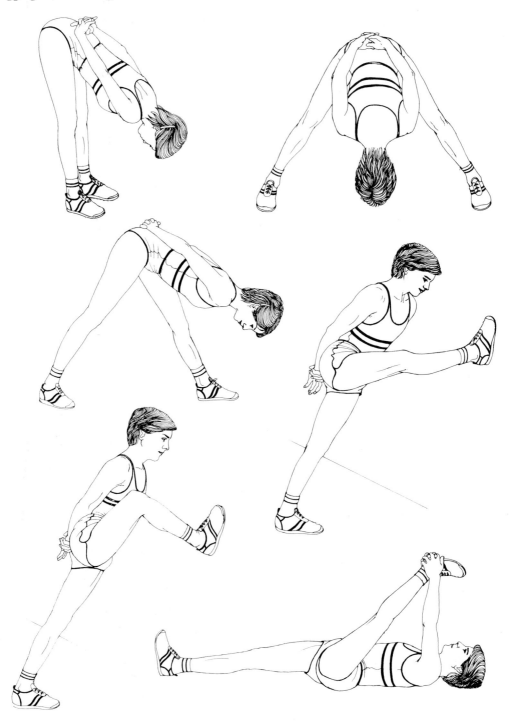

Cycling

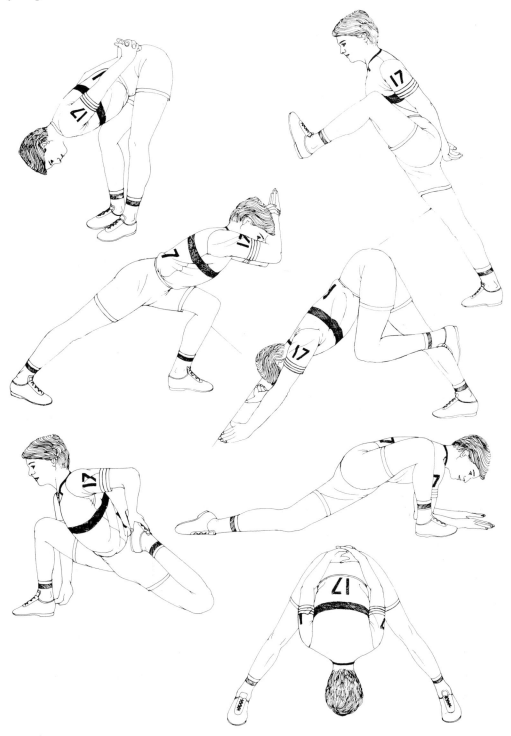

Tennis, Squash and Badminton

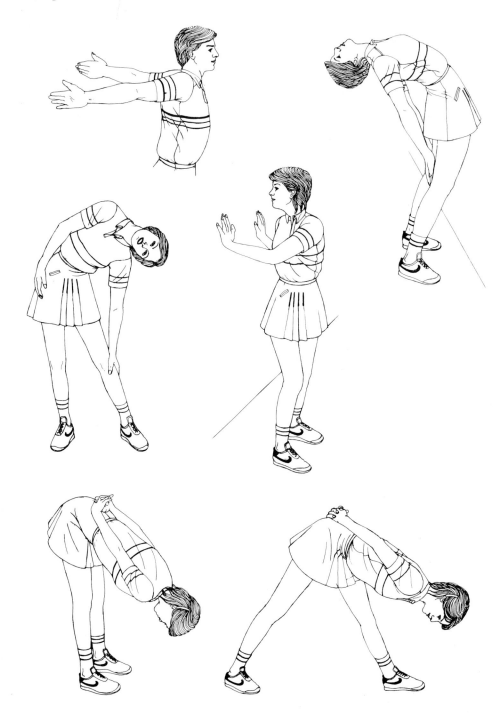

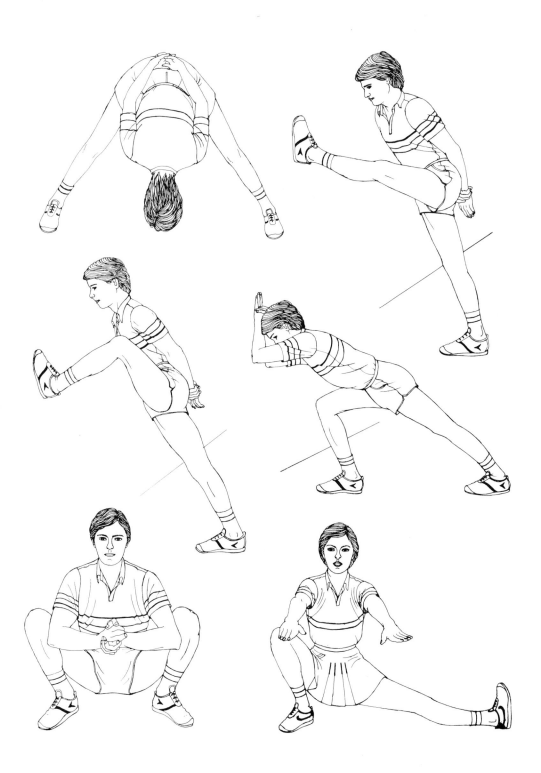

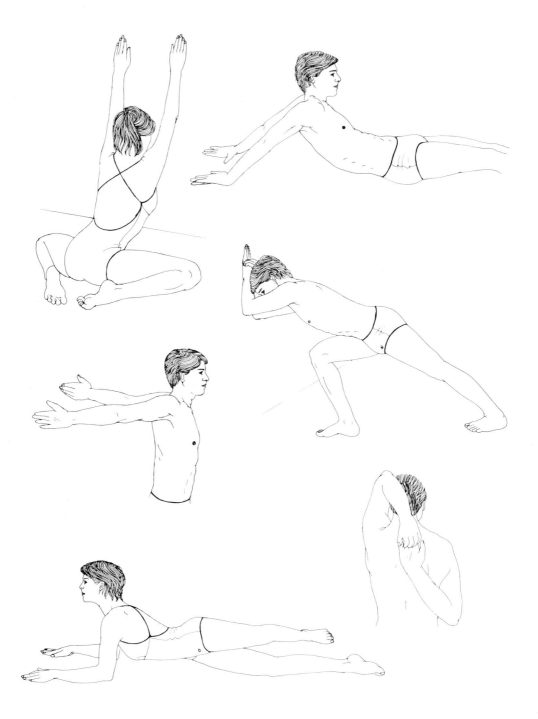

Golf

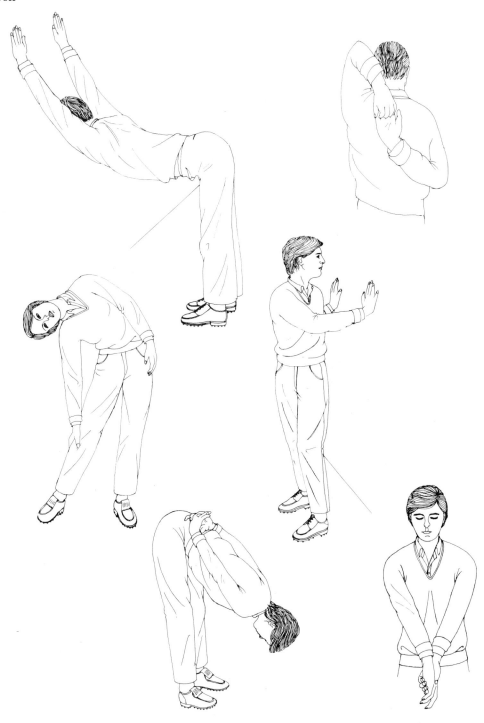

Skiing

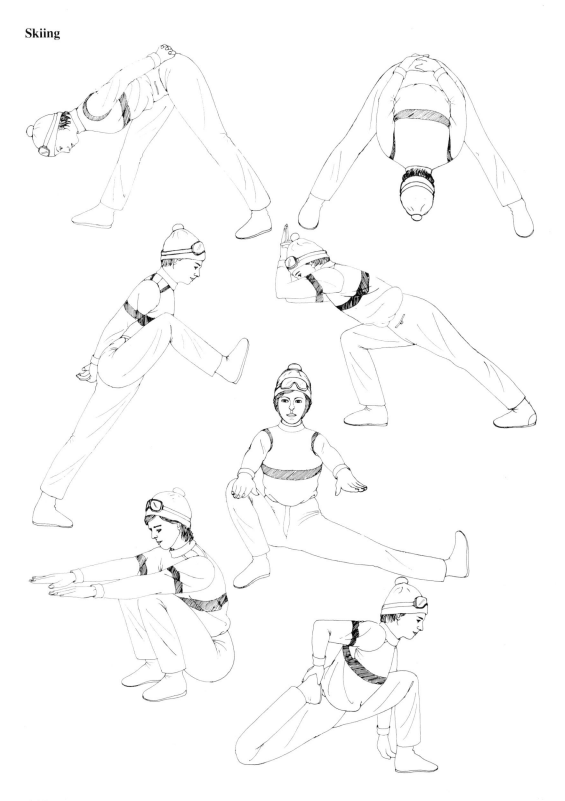

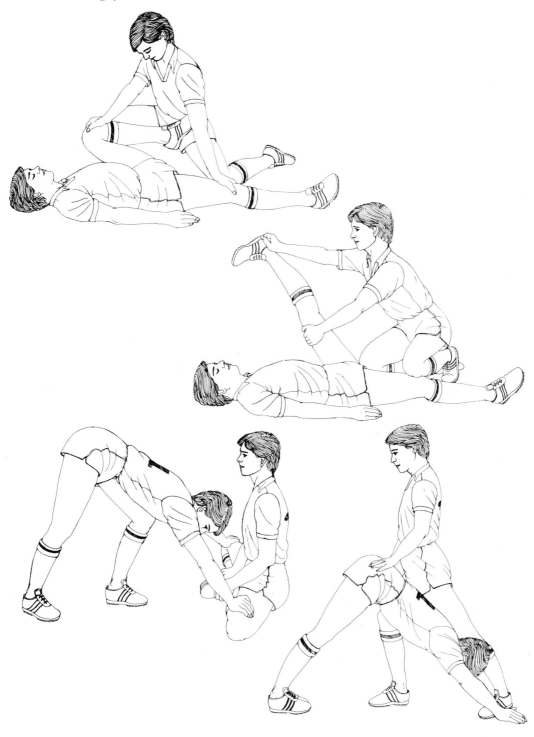

119

Cricket

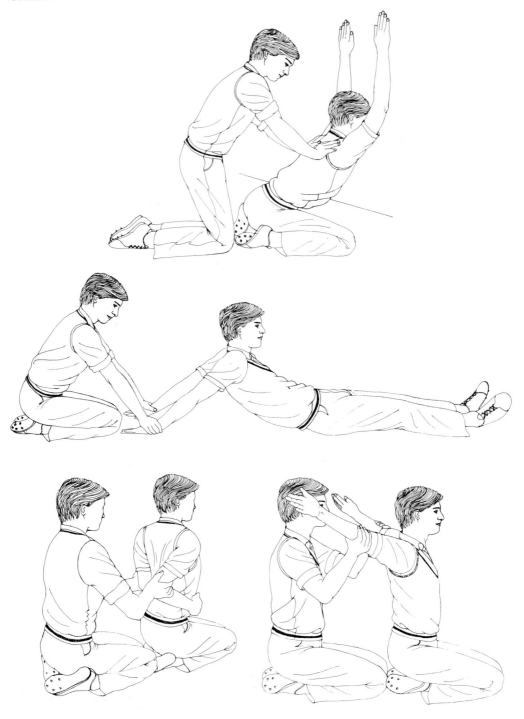

Baseball

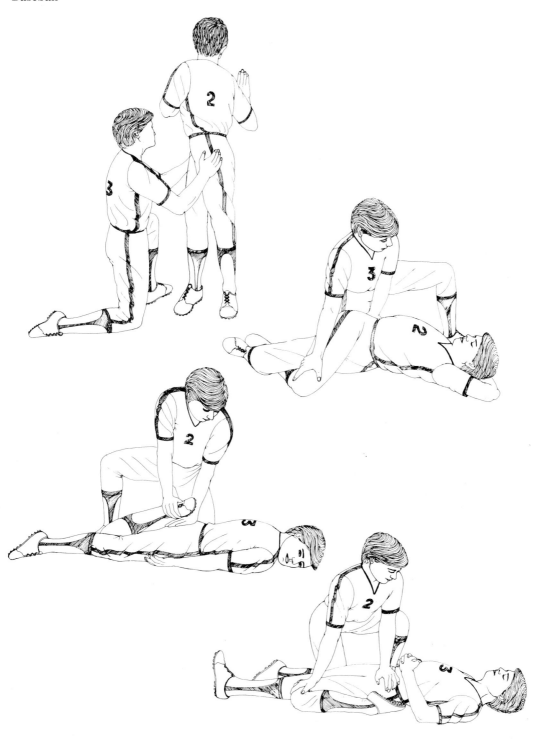

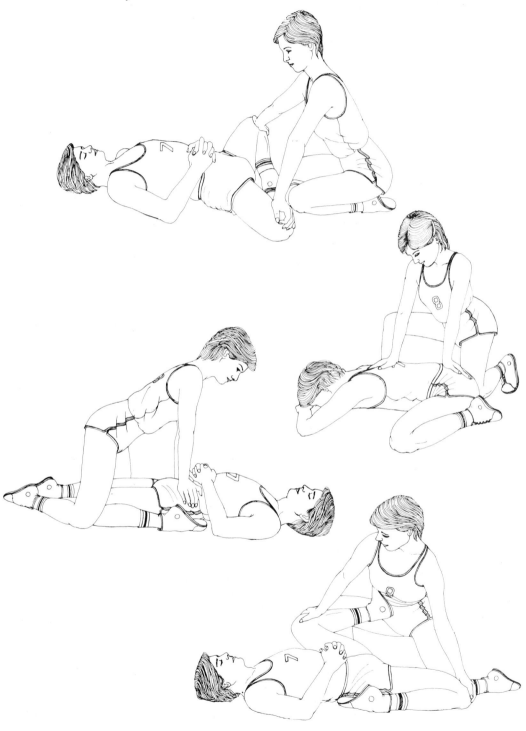

10. Stretching for Martial Arts, Yoga and Meditation

Martial Arts

If you practise any of the martial arts, tai-chi, akido, kempo, karate, judo, kung-fu and so on, suppleness is an essential component towards being successful in that art. An akido master once said that the difference between a great martial artist and a competent one was their degree of effortless flexibility. He was commenting on how many western students had stiff backs. The effortless action demanded by the martial arts of China and Japan can never be reached without full flexibility and elasticity at every joint and muscle. Practising any martial art with a stiff or partially stiff body is like playing a musical instrument that is slightly out of tune. The following stretches are recommended as a supplement for anyone practising any martial art.

Yoga

The classical *asanas* or postures of yoga may be divided into two groups. The first consists of positions that are assisted by gravity, like the standing forward bend (*uttinasana*), the tailor position (*buddhakanasana*), and the lotus (*padmasana*), which is the most essential position because it is used as the foundation for yogic breathing exercises (*pranayama*) and meditation (*dyana*). The second group are balancing positions like the head stand (*sirsasana*) and shoulder stand (*sarangasana*) which are traditionally considered the mother and father of all *asanas*. The first group involves positions that demand extreme ranges of movement at various joints and extreme stretches of muscles and tendons. The emphasis of the second group on the other hand emphasises defying gravity and proper alignment of the body.

If you practise yoga all the partner stretches of chapter 7 plus the following stretches are recommended. These are preliminary and complementary positions that are not classically yogic but aid you in achieving the classic *asanas* of yoga.

Meditation

Stretching to be able to sit in the lotus position

Most meditation and breathing practice involves sitting positions of some kind. The ultimate classical position for these practices is the 'lotus' with an effortless balanced head and trunk. The 'awareness (*satipatthana*) discourse of the Buddha' is one of the earliest Pali texts, and considered by most Buddhists to be the essence of their whole meditation practice. In its very first instruction on awareness of breathing it refers to sitting down. It says, 'Having gone to the forest to the foot of a tree or to an empty place, one sits down crossed legged, keeps one's body erect and one's awareness alert. Thus with awareness one breathes in and out'. For most of us today sitting down for any length of time with crossed legs and an effortlessly balanced trunk is not easy. The lotus position may be divided into two parts, the legs as the base and the trunk and head as the balanced upright. Being able to sit with your legs crossed is only the first step and any stiffness in the hips, knees and ankles makes this very difficult. The second step is even more difficult, that is balancing your trunk and head in perfect alignment. This is only possible when every joint of your trunk, neck and shoulders is fully flexible. Your trunk and head can never balance effortlessly until your spine can bend backwards, forwards and sideways fully.

In other words you cannot sit perfectly upright with ease if your trunk is stiff. Trying to do so just creates more tension and stiffness. The first step to the lotus is the base which demands flexion and outward rotation of your hips and knees. The second step demands all-round flexibility. The stretches of chapter 6 include specific stretches for crossing the legs and for making all the major joints of the body flexible. There are other positions that can be used as alternatives by people who are unable to assume the lotus. They still involve sitting with a balanced trunk and head, with flexed hips and knees for some length of time.

Stretches after sitting in any position for a long time
The following stretches are recommended for after you have been sitting for long periods of time in any position, whether for meditation or for breathing exercises or for anything else.

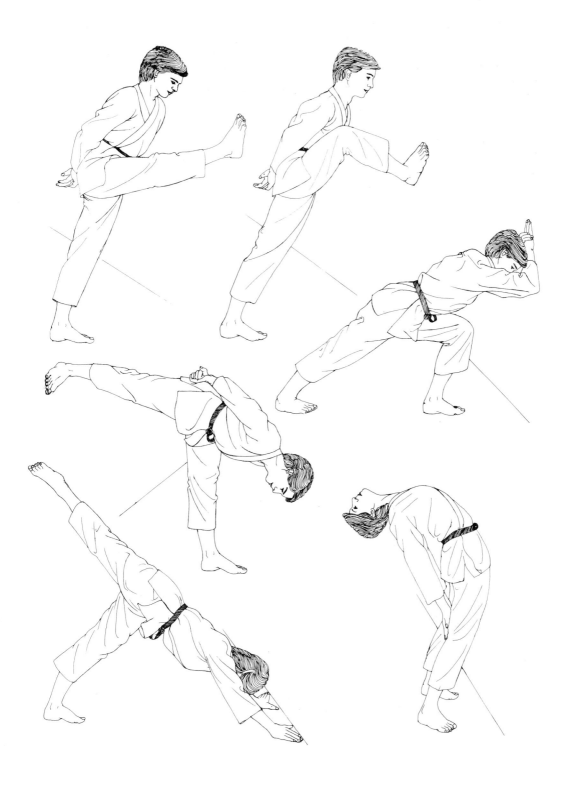

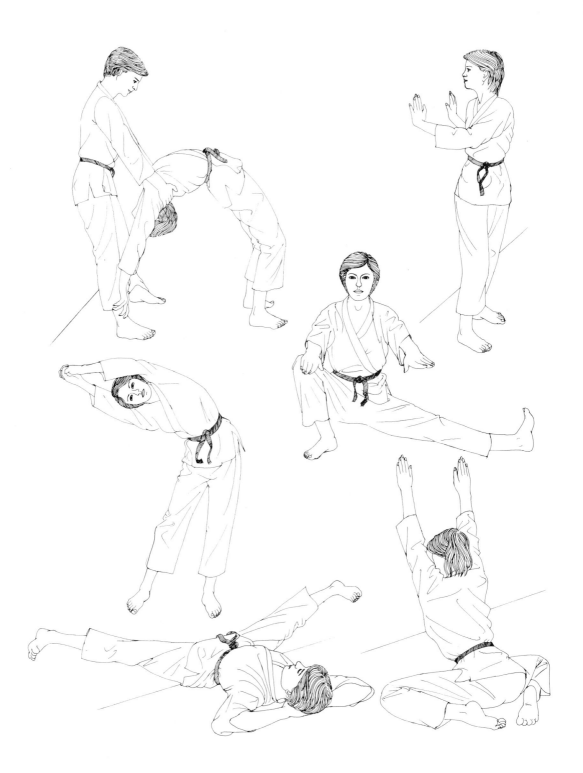

126

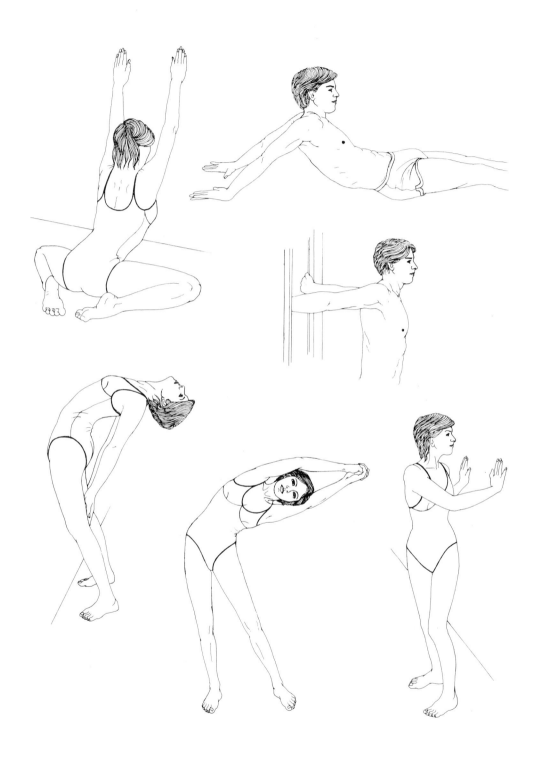

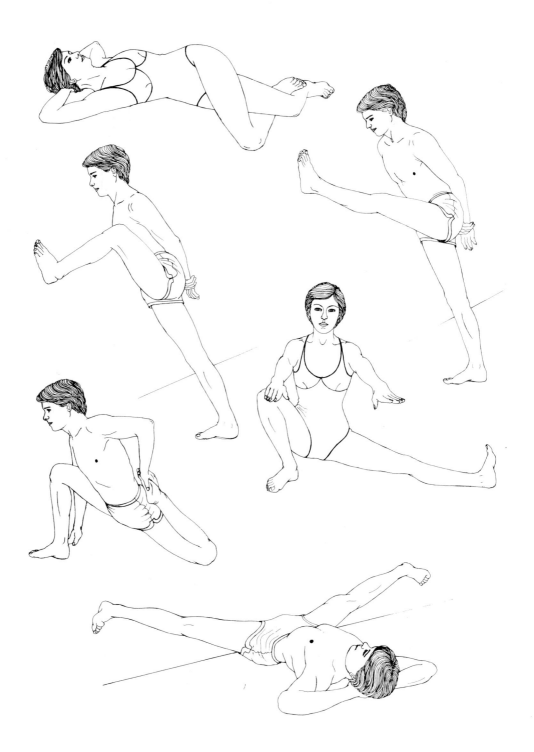

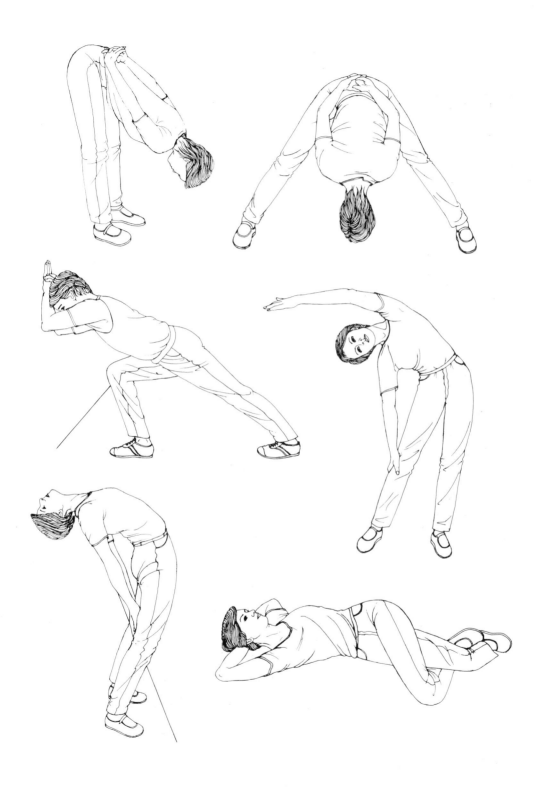

129

11. Stretching and Childbirth

Pregnancy begins at conception and is the time in which a child grows and develops until it is ready to be born. Perhaps at no other time in a woman's life is stretching regularly needed more. Her baby's health depends on her health. Stretching makes her body's musculo-skeletal system supple and fit. During this time a variety of hormones flow into a woman's bloodstream causing her joints, muscles, tendons and ligaments to become more supple. Stretching during pregnancy further promotes their suppleness and merely takes full advantage of nature's preparation. If any of a woman's joints are stiff she needs to improve her ability to stretch and relax the muscles governing them. However, the pelvis together with the area immediately above and below it is the part of her body that should be made as supple and relaxable as possible for giving birth. When a woman stretches a group of muscles she is relaxing them, furthermore, she increases their ability in the future to relax in action. The fit of her child's head in her pelvis is so exact that the smallest increase in the size of her pelvic opening during labour is significant. At this time she needs flexible pelvic walls. She will have made her child's passage through her birth canal easier if she has properly stretched her pelvic joints and their muscles during pregnancy, so allowing her to position her pelvis at its widest when giving birth.

For a woman to be able to move and change her bodily position during labour is a natural, instinctive response that should be open to her. She should feel free to stand, squat, lie, kneel, walk, in fact, assume any comfortable position which can assist the task of her uterus and the muscles of her birth canal. This response is more available to a woman if she has been stretching regularly during pregnancy.

The type of exercises suitable for pregnancy must be non-strenuous, neither straining nor tiring. They should save energy and release tension; reduce a woman's heartbeat and breathing rate; and always be assisted by gravity rather than resisted by it. Stretching fits all these demands. Through the various stretches a woman gently and gradually and powerfully encourages her joints and muscles to give up their habitual stiffness. Some stretches may be done while having a bath, others just before going to sleep; some may be done at any time and others need a set time each day when she won't be disturbed.

As stretching regularly balances the opposing muscle-powers which govern joints, it adjusts and improves posture automatically without making one self-conscious of posture. During the last months of pregnancy a woman carries an extra load – her growing baby. Perhaps at no other time is it more beneficial to have a properly balanced posture or is it more essential to improve it as much as possible.

Stretching regularly during pregnancy directs a woman's attention to her body. This subtly changes her feeling of her physical self. It doesn't make her self-conscious. What it does is increase her self-awareness. All the benefits of practising stretching, that is, improved suppleness, posture, relaxation, breathing, circulation, and energy are especially desirable during this vital time.

The obvious benefit is the ability to use a number of natural birth positions.

By stretching regularly during pregnancy, squatting, kneeling or other natural birth postures will not be unfamiliar or difficult when the day of birth begins. A woman can by practising stretching exercises increase the mobility of her pelvis. Giving birth is fundamentally a physical feat and like any physical feat no one could expect to be successful without some preparation, study and above all, practise of the positions necessary to perform the feat

130

most easily. Stretching regularly is a wonderful preparation for labour and childbirth. The point of physical preparation is to get the muscles of a woman's body especially those of her lower trunk in the best condition during the months before labour begins.

Regular practise of the soft stretching exercises of chapters 6 and 7 naturally prepares a woman's body to be at its best for her pregnancy and her child's birth (and it helps her to recover quickly afterwards).

However, once you are pregnant there comes a time when not all the stretches are to be practised any more. At this point a specific series of stretches is needed and appropriate – those positions that open your pelvis, thighs and pelvic floor. These include many positions like squatting and kneeling that are instinctively natural to use during labour and childbirth.

Very soon after giving birth there comes a time when you are able and ready to start stretching again. At this point another series of stretches is appropriate – those positions that close the pelvis and particularly the pelvic floor. Several months later you can then resume regular practise of the stretches of chapters 6 and 7.

Summary of Stages
1. Before you become pregnant – stretches of chapters 6 and 7.
2. When pregnant the following stretches are recommended, many of which can be used during labour and birth.
3. Shortly after the birth the following stretches are recommended most of which close and strengthen the floor of the pelvis.
4. Several months afterwards – the stretches of chapters 6 and 7 again.

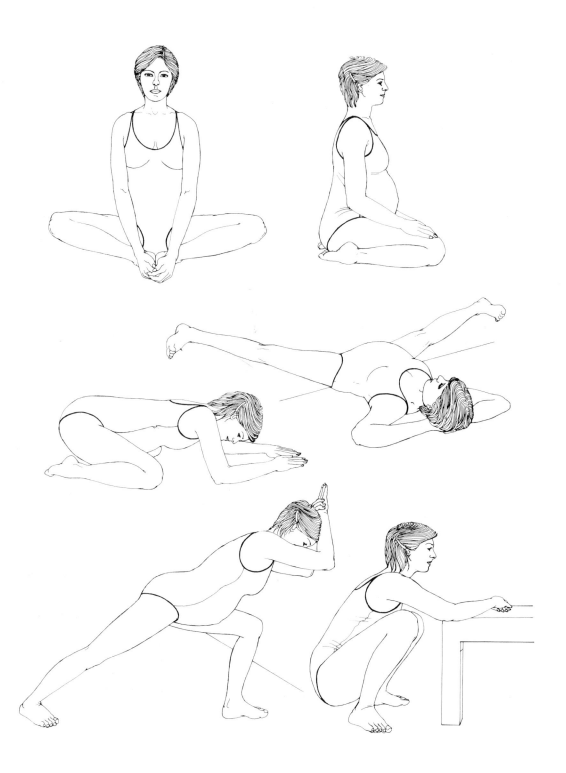

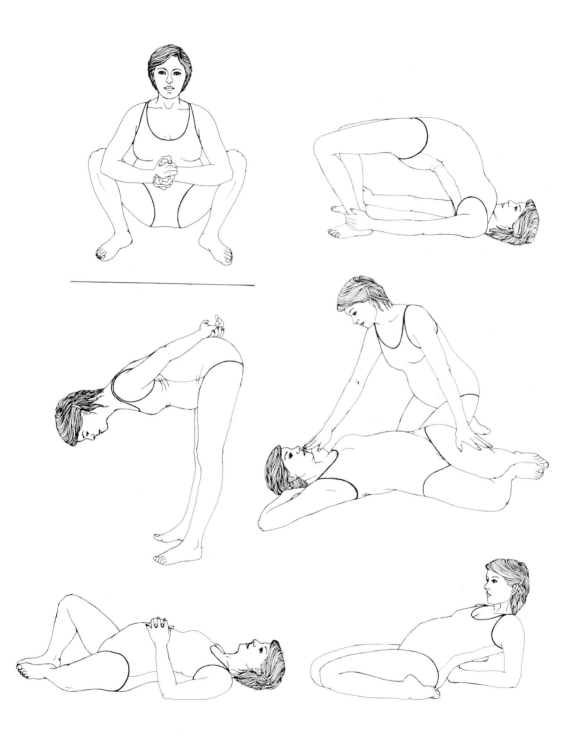

133

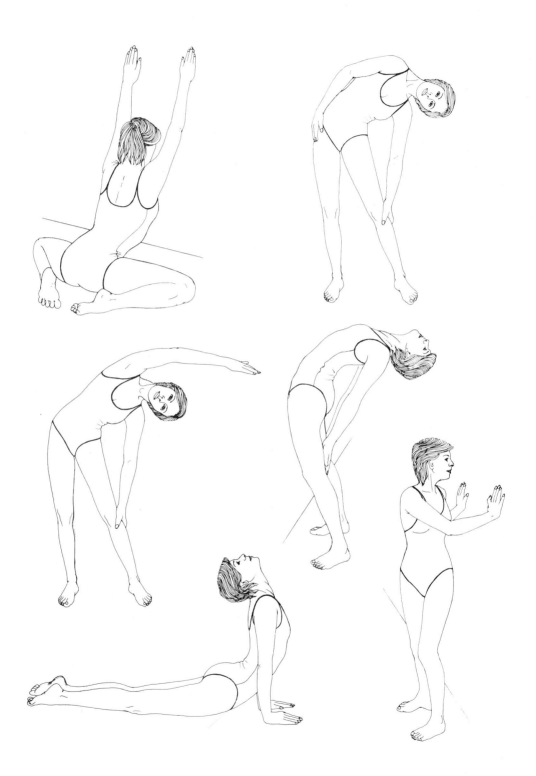

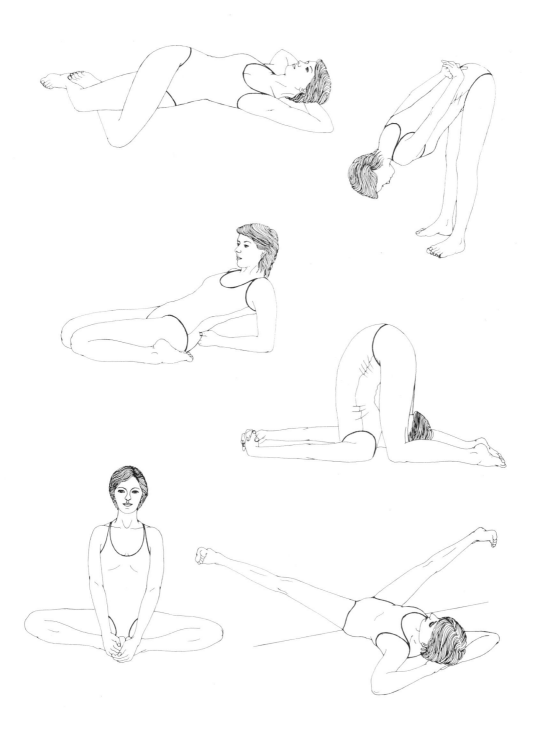

12. Stretching and Physical Education

Why do most of us become stiff from about the age of five onwards? Why do our joints gradually lose their flexibility and our muscles their elasticity when we get older? Why does only one in every five people escape arthritic and rheumatic pain problems by the age of sixty? Why do eight out of ten people on earth at some point in their lives suffer from back pain? Obviously because of the wear and tear of life, because of the traumas and pains of living. But why does stiffening seem to happen so quickly and why – if regular stretching avoids this and is so important for the health of one's musculo-skeletal system– do so few people practise this good habit? The answer to this is poor physical education, the kind of physical education that most of us get at school. Most schools encourage games and sports but very little worthwhile physical education. The average PE class lays stress on endurance and strength. While stretching is almost non-existent. The antidote to the eventual wear and tear of life is the proper physical education that comes from stretching regularly from the first school year to the last.

Whether you excel in sports and games or not, you should learn at school how to take care of your body's musculo-skeletal system yourself. After all school is supposed to prepare you for life. You should learn that you cannot depend on other people to take care of your body's joints and muscles and that to be in the best of health your body should be supple. Throughout the school years a child should learn that stretching is the simplest and most effective way of relaxing the body. That stretching improves the rate and depth of breathing, increases blood and lymph circulation, takes a load off the heart and contributes to the body's defence against harmful agents. That stretching improves one of the major senses of the mind – your muscle sense (proprioception) – your very awareness of your physical self. That the anatomy one learns through stretching comes from your own body through direct perception. That stretching improves the operation of the will – the more flexible your body the greater command you have over it. That stretching changes the bodily frame – by improving the function of the joints and muscles and naturally improves posture, form and beauty. That consistent stretching brings an overall feeling of lightness and energy. That stretching adds to opening up physical armour and the blocked emotions behind it.

At school you should learn how to keep your body from becoming old before its time and free from headaches, backaches, arthritis and rheumatism. That stretching, not only before activity or before and after long periods of sitting, but anytime we felt like it, would improve our physical health and enjoyment of movement and activity a lot more.

Usually at school there are two mainstreams of pupils, those that get into sports and dance and those that have no aptitude for physical games and so drop out of effectively using their bodies during their critical school years. Whichever group a child belongs to, or wherever he or she comes between those two groups, to avoid arthritis and rheumatism in later life stretching should be encouraged through school as a daily physical practice to be continued for the rest of one's life. Any child leaving school stiff is, in effect, going into the world with a body that is partially paralysed and partially dislocated. These are strong terms, but true. As no child should leave school without the ability to read and write so no child should leave school without a supple healthy body free from stiffness at every joint. Stretching daily at school lays the foundations for a healthy musculo-skeletal system for the rest of life and should be so taught that it becomes a second nature activity.

136

50,000 people a day suffer from back pain and 18 million working days are lost each year in Great Britain. As a result 900 million pounds are lost to British Industry and 90 million pounds paid out by social security each year. In America 75 million people have back problems and back pain claims 7 million new victims each year of which 5 million are partially disabled and 2 million unable to work at all. 93 million working days are lost each year in the USA as a result of back pain and the Americans spend 5 billion dollars a year on tests and treatment. In Sweden the largest single cause of absenteeism from work is back pain and 25 per cent of people retiring from work before their time do so as a result of this universal affliction.

Some Suggested Stretching Routines

Here are some basic stretch routines for everyone. There are routines for the stiff beginner, standard routines for those with an average degree of flexibility and routines for the very flexible. There is also a special routine for getting what we call the deep stretch. Within each category of routine are programmes of different length. Your choice will obviously depend on how much time you have or want to spend on stretching at any given time. It is advisable to try the easy routines first and move onto the others when you feel that you are ready. Remember there is no rush, in fact you cannot rush the cultivation of flexibility. Your muscles and joints will not allow it. It may take months and years to graduate to the final stretches. But every time you stretch you are making progress and getting the benefits that stretching gives you, however stiff or supple you may be. Feel your way, there are no hard and fast rules. Once you are stretching regularly you will develop routines to suit yourself, the given routines are not obligatory. Stretch to suit your body and your own particular circumstances.

Some Beginner Stretch Routines
The fact that you are beginning or stiff may present a challenge. But the stiffer you are you will reap the greatest benefits as there is so much to gain. The only contest is between you and your muscles and joints – no one else.

A five-minute routine for beginners

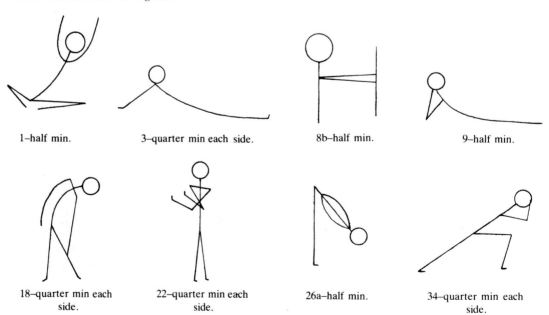

1–half min.   3–quarter min each side.   8b–half min.   9–half min.

18–quarter min each side.   22–quarter min each side.   26a–half min.   34–quarter min each side.

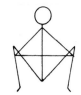

36–quarter min. 42a–quarter min. 45a–quarter min. 55–quarter min.

A fifteen-minute routine for beginners

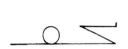 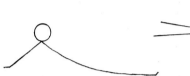 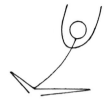

1–half min. 2–half min. 3–half min palms up, half min palms down. 8a–half min.

8b–half min. 4a–quarter min each side. 4b–quarter min each side. 6–half min each side.

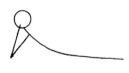 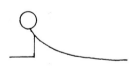 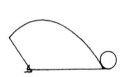 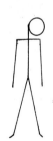

9–half min. 10–half min. 15–half min. 17–quarter min each side.

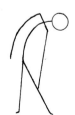 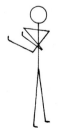

18–half min each side. 21–quarter min each side. 22–quarter min each side. 24–half min.

139

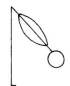 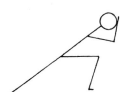 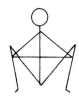

26a–half min.   34–quarter min each side.   36–half min.   42a–half min.

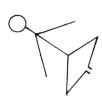 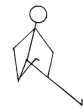 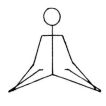

43–half min.   45a–half min.   47–quarter min each side.   49a–half min.

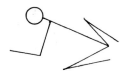 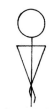

50a–half min.   54–quarter min each   55–half min.
                 side.

A half-hour routine for beginners

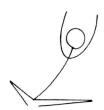 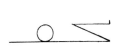 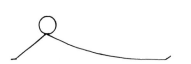

1–one min.   2–one min.   3–half min each side.   4a–quarter min
                                                      each side.

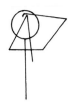 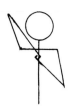 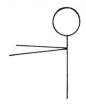

4b–quarter min
each side.

6–quarter min
each side.

7–quarter min
each side.

8a–half min.

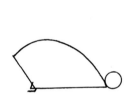 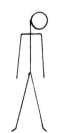 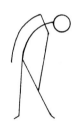 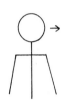

8b–half min.

9–one min.

10–one min.

11–half min each side.

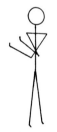 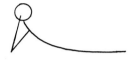 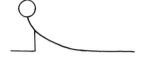 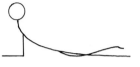

15–half min.

17–quarter min each side.

18–half min each side.

21–quarter min each side.

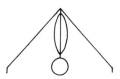 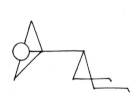

22–half min each side.

23–half min each side.

26a–half min each side.

26b–half min each side.

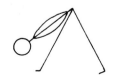 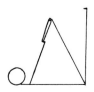 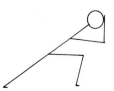

27–one min.

28–half min each side.

32a–half min each side.

34–half min each side.

141

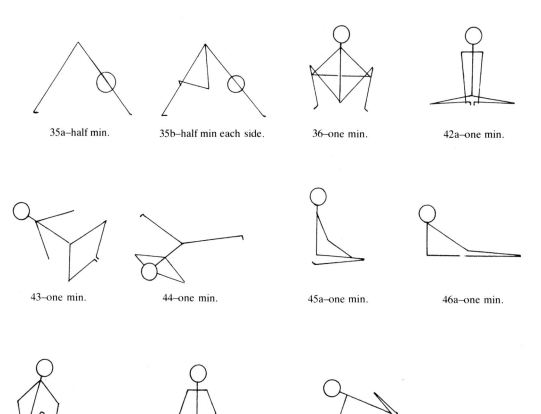

35a–half min. 35b–half min each side. 36–one min. 42a–one min.

43–one min. 44–one min. 45a–one min. 46a–one min.

47–half min each side. 49a–one min. 50a–half min.

For a one-hour beginners routine simply double all the timings.

Some Intermediate Routines

These stretch routines will take you further than the beginning stretches. If you possess average flexibility that is somewhere between quite stiff and very flexible they are ideal. Practising these intermediate stretches will keep you loose and relaxed and will gradually lead you into the more advanced stretches.

A five-minute intermediate routine

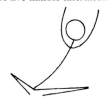 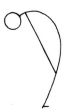 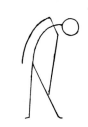

1–half min. 7–quarter min each side. 12–half min. 18–quarter min each side.

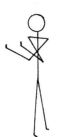

22–quarter min
each side.

26a–half min.

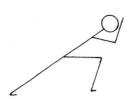

34–quarter min each side.

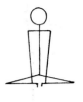

42a–half min.

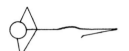

46b–half min.

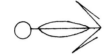

50b–half min.

A fifteen-minute intermediate routine

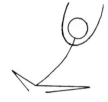

1–one min.

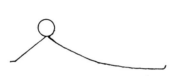

3–half min each side.

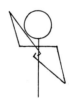

7–half min each side.

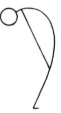

12–one min.

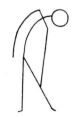

18–half min each side.

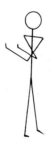

22–half min each side.

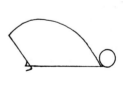

25–one min.

26a–one min.

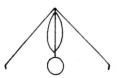

27–one min.

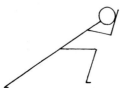

34–half min each side.

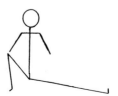

38–half min each side.

42a–one min.

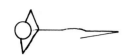

46b–one min.

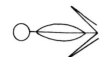

50b–one min.

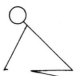

55–one min.

A forty-five minute intermediate routine

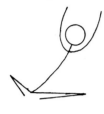

1–one min.

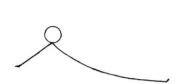

3–one min each side.

4a–quarter min each side.

4b–quarter min each side.

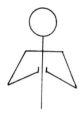

5–half min.

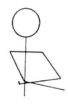

6–quarter min each side.

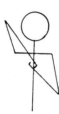

7–half min each side.

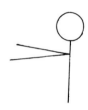

8a–half min.

8b–one min.

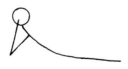

9–one min.

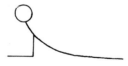

10–one min.

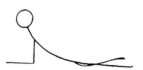

11–half min each side.

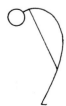

12–half min.

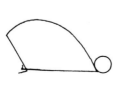

15–half min.

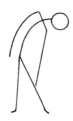

18–half min each side.

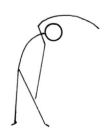

19–half min each side.

144

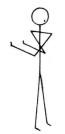 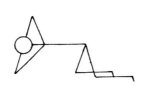 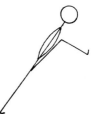

22–half min each side.   23–half min each side.   25–one min.   26a–one min.

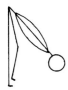 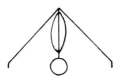 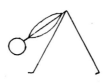 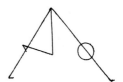

26b–half min each side.   27–one min.   28–half min each side.   30–half min each side.

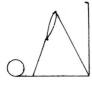 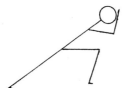 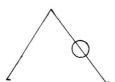

32a–half min each side.   34–one min each side.   35a–one min.   35b–half min each side.

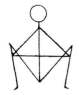 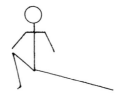 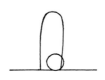

36–one min.   37a–half min.   38–quarter min each side.   39–half min.

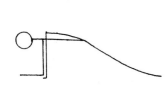 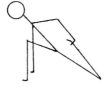 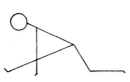 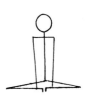

40a–half min each side.   40b–quarter min each side.   41a–half min.   42a–2 mins.

145

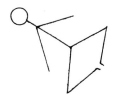 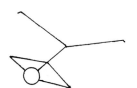 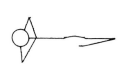

43–2 mins.   44–one and a half mins.   45a–2 mins.   46b–one min.

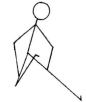 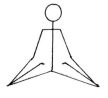 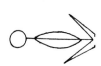 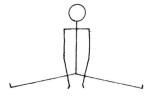

47–half min each side.   49a–one min.   50b–one min.   51–one min.

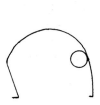 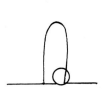

54–quarter min each side.   55–one min.

Some routines for the Very Flexible

These routines emphasise extreme movement. Once you start becoming really supple they should suit you perfectly. It takes time to get to this stage. But by the time you are there you will really appreciate the enormous benefits and the subtleties of a flexible, supple body. At this stage your body will feel so alive it will literally sing to you. Once you reach these final stretches you just need to maintain your full range of movement by regular practice.

A five-minute routine for the very flexible

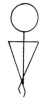 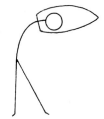 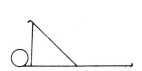

16–half min.   20–quarter min each side.   25–half min.   32b–quarter min each side.

146

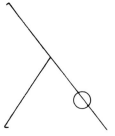 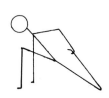 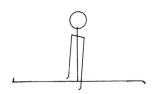

35c–quarter min each side. 40b–quarter min each side.   41b–quarter min each side.   42b–half min.

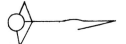 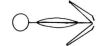 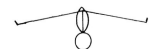

46b–half min. 50b–quarter min. 53–quarter min.

A fifteen-minute routine for the very flexible

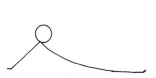 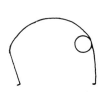 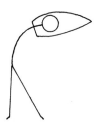

3–half min palms up, half min   7–quarter min   16–half min.   20–quarter min
palms down.   each side.   each side.

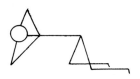 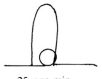 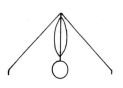

23–half min each side.   25–one min.   26a–half min.   27–half min.

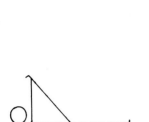

32b–half min each side.

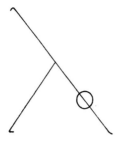

35c–half min each side.

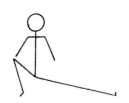

38–half min each side.

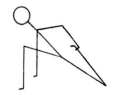

40b–half min each side.

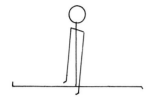

41b–half min each side.

42b–half min.

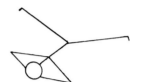

44–one min.

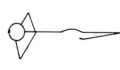

46b–half min.

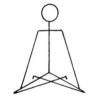

48–half min each side.

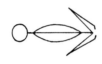

50b–half min.

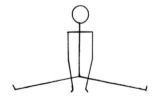

51–quarter min each side.

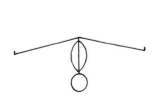

53–half min.

55–half min.

148

A sixty-minute routine for the very flexible

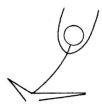

1–one min.

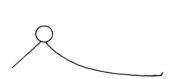

3–one min palms up, one min palms down.

5–one min.

7–one min each side.

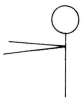

8b–one min.

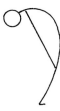

12–one min.

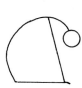

13–one min.

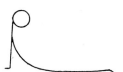

14–one min.

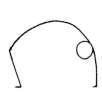

16–one min.

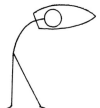

20–half min each side.

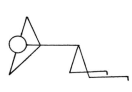

23–one min each side.

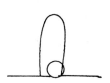

25–two mins.

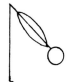

26a–one min.

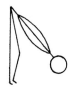

26b–one min each side.

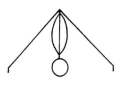

27–two mins.

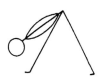

28–one min each side.

149

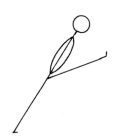 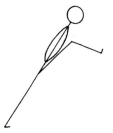 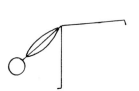 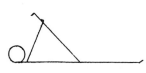

29–one min each side.   30–one min each side.   31–one min each side.   32b–one min each side.

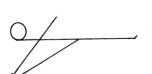 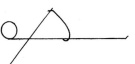 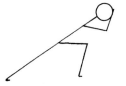 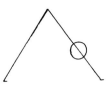

33a–half min each side.   33b–half min each side.   34–one min each side.   35a–one min.

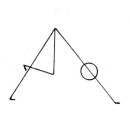 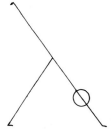 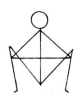 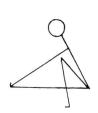

35b–half min each side.   35c–half min each side.   36–one min.   37b–half min each side.

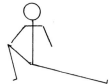 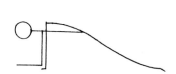

38–half min each side.   39–half min.   40a–half min each side.   40b–half min each side.

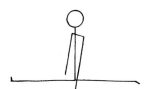   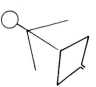

41b–half min each side.   42a–two mins.   42b–one min.   43–two mins.

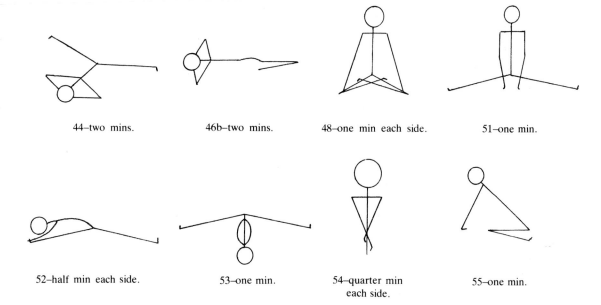

44–two mins.　　46b–two mins.　　48–one min each side.　　51–one min.

52–half min each side.　　53–one min.　　54–quarter min each side.　　55–one min.

The deep stretch routine

This routine is for those who love to stretch or for those who have discovered how stiff they really are, are challenged by it and would really like to make rapid and sudden progress.

This routine will find its way deep into your muscle tissue and will enable you to experience sensations that you have probably never felt before. This routine demands perseverance, staying power, and the ability to let go. It need only be practised at most once or twice a week. You need no particular prowess. It is perfectly safe. Stretching deeply at this level simply involves lying around in resting stretching positions for longer periods of time.

These are the positions in which one can spend longer time. You may chose any combination of these stretches depending on how much time you have.

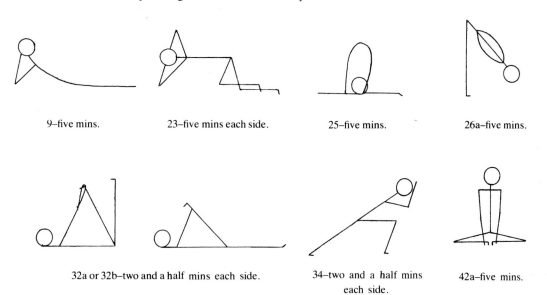

9–five mins.　　23–five mins each side.　　25–five mins.　　26a–five mins.

32a or 32b–two and a half mins each side.　　34–two and a half mins each side.　　42a–five mins.

151

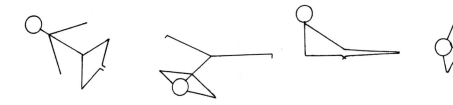

43–five mins.   44–five mins.   46a or 46b–five mins.

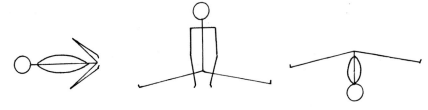

50b–five mins.   51 or 53–five mins.